MOO VET

One Veterinarian's Role in Food Supply and Sustaining Humanity

Samuel P. Galphin DVM, MS

Published by SuburbanBuzz.com LLC

ISBN: 978-1-959446-19-4

DEDICATION

I could not have written this manuscript without the help of some special people, the chief of whom is my wife, Shelley. Truth be known, she has tolerated my crazy hours, my frustrations, my excitements, and especially my absences for almost 50 years as I drove and flew around the globe. Without her support and tolerance, I could never have been an effective food supply veterinarian and dairyman. People suspect that we are given angels at times to help us along in our life journey. Shelley is mine. She allowed me to follow my passion for feeding people, which, in turn, gave me the food for this book. Thank you, Shelley, for your love and immense contributions to my life!

CONTENTS

ACKNOWLEDGMENTS

I would be negligent not to acknowledge the many mentors I have had during my career. A mentor is defined as "an experienced and trusted advisor or someone who trains and counsels, especially a younger colleague." I will not bore you with their roles, but I want to recognize them by name for the time they invested in me. I will understandably start with my dad and mom, both departed now. Then I must mention my children, for whom among us doesn't learn life lessons from their children.

Great organizations like Christian Veterinary Mission (cvmusa.org) should be acknowledged for spreading veterinary science and the gospel of Jesus Christ. Heifer Project International (heifer.org) and Freedom Global (freedomglobal.org), also, are commended for helping to end hunger, poverty, and illiteracy.

Lastly, I list the most influential of my professional associates and connections: Dr. Fred Trout, Dr. Eberhard Rosin, Dr. Tom Randolph, Mr. Bill McGee, Dr. Ben Harrington, Dr. Ben Shelton, Dr. Jim Nash, Dr. Livio Feruzzi, Dr. Page Wages, Dr. Mike Gilsdorf, Mr. Douglas Child, Mr. David Falk, Mr. Alvis Fleming, Mr. Fred Jaques, Mr. Greg Langley and Mr. Weathers. Of course, there are many others, too numerous to count, and I thank you all immensely.

INTRODUCTION
A Journey into Food Supply Veterinary Medicine

Growing up on a farm in rural South Carolina instilled in me a sound work ethic, a love of nature, and a love of agriculture. By the time I graduated from high school, I was sure that I wanted to be a veterinarian just like my dad, who was a rural mixed animal practitioner. In college, I was pressed to excel academically by the struggle to pay for my own education, a very low military draft number, and the Vietnam conflict. Therefore, I rapidly moved through undergraduate school at Clemson University and into veterinary school at the University of Georgia.

While at veterinary school, I kept my student military draft deferral active until my junior year, when I applied for and received an armed forces scholarship. This scholarship reduced my monetary and academic pressures, but it committed me to two years of active military service after graduation. This, in fact, was okay with me because as I approached graduation, I began to realize that I would not be happy back in rural South Carolina in my dad's mixed animal practice. The military commitment allowed me to postpone that conversation with my dad.

I remember returning home during a school break in my second year of veterinary school. Dad asked me to go on an emergency call with him. We examined a cow in respiratory distress, and he asked me what my diagnosis was and how I would treat it. Now at that point in my studies, I had only been exposed to basic sciences like anatomy, chemistry, and physiology. No diseases had ever been discussed. Proudly, seeing his desire to have me be a part of his practice, I responded that I thought the animal had Hemorrhagic Septicemia, treatable by injectable antibiotics. He looked confusedly at me and

1

concurred with my diagnosis. I don't know where that disease diagnosis came from in my brain because when I got home, I had to look up what it was.

Hemorrhagic Septicemia is a respiratory disease caused by a specific Pasteurella bacteria and is treatable with antibiotics. However, it is mainly seen in cattle and goats in South America. My dad had concurred with my diagnosis, perhaps because he had never heard of Hemorrhagic Septicemia. Or, perhaps when he had studied veterinary medicine 40 years earlier, all respiratory disease was called Hemorrhagic Septicemia since the sophisticated serological test that identified the specific Pasteurella organism was not yet discovered. Nonetheless, Dad acted satisfied, and I never had the courage to ask him what he really thought about the diagnosis.

Secretly, I began to wonder if his type of practice, working on a variety of individual animals, was the type of practice that I would enjoy. This attitude allowed me not to have any preconceived ideas of what I would do after veterinary school, and as a result, I availed myself of every opportunity to learn everything I could while I was in veterinary college. I joined every clinical course offered outside of the usual required surgeries, medicines, and "ology's," including subjects like laboratory animal medicine, caged bird medicine, and a new course called herd health medicine.

Throughout my veterinary education, I was exposed to the biases of the various faculty members. The companion animal faculty members preached that their disciplines allowed vets to practice the challenging "real" medicine, similar to human practice, with all its scientific diagnostic aids. The companion animal faculty derided the food animal practitioner as unscientific and arcane. The food animal medicine faculty extolled the virtues of the outdoors, the excitement of motoring through the countryside, and the relationships built with the livestock farmers when one endeavors to prevent losses in their livestock.

Nevertheless, neither of these camps captured my exclusive attention. During my senior year in vet school, I began to realize that I wanted to do more than just work on animals; I wanted to give back to mankind in some way through my work in the veterinary profession. I was young and idealistic, as most youth are. I was especially moved by a quote of Mark Twain, "The two greatest days of your life are the day you were born and the day you find out why."

Purpose in life to me was far more important than possessions. Having more to live with was no substitute for having more to live for. I recognized that I could have a role in the essential area of food production or feeding the world, but I also aspired to find ways to involve myself in the exciting field of comparative research where my training could be more directly applied to human problems. I was fortunate during my senior year to be able to collaborate with a vet school faculty member and participate in his research projects. The ensuing mentorship resulted in my being included as an author on three publications on human comparative medical topics before I even graduated. This work paid off later when I entered academia after military service.

I was sure that comparative medicine was my thing until I enrolled in that senior-level course in herd health medicine, now referred to as production medicine or food supply veterinary medicine. The instructor was a visionary in many ways. He applied veterinary medicine to animal production and aptly demonstrated the many challenges of producing a profit while producing food. He was able to apply economics to almost every aspect of food supply veterinary medicine, and it all seemed so logical and exciting to me. He demonstrated to us, his students, the effects that the animal's environment had on animal health and productivity, and he challenged us to find answers to problems that we never thought were problems.

Traditional veterinary education at that time steered us to assume our role was diagnosing and treating individual animals sickened by diseases. It did not relate our training to other biological processes critical to food production profitability. The professor in this course showed us that our training prepared us for a more "holistic" approach to animal health, which included not only the known diseases but also a myriad of other factors that affect animal health and productivity. He showed us how air flow, temperature, nutrition, housing, management, and other environmental properties influence the health and productivity of livestock.

This professor's visionary approach destroyed the companion animal faculty's assertion that food supply veterinary medicine was unscientific and arcane. Moreover, during my senior year, I was drawn to a local church in Athens, Georgia, doing a study series on the world food situation. The study was both exhilarating and depressing at the same time. I realized that I could find purpose in food supply

3

veterinary medicine. By graduation, I was intent on making food supply veterinary medicine my career choice.

Nonetheless, "Uncle Sam" reminded me I owed a debt to my country after graduation, and I was called to serve two years in the United States Air Force. I was not sent to Vietnam because America withdrew forces from there during my senior year. My admiration and respect go out to those who were called into service during that terrible conflict. The Air Force sent me to Columbus, Mississippi, to an Air Training Command base. This base had the mission to train young pilots. My military duties were primarily focused on human food safety but also included human disease monitoring and traceability as I assumed the dual role of bio-environmental science officer and veterinary officer.

I found a special opportunity in the Air Force when I was allowed to conduct some airbase-level research. I applied for and was funded by the Department of Defense for a comparative research project on the zoonotic disease, Brucella canis. A zoonotic disease is passed from animals to humans. The importance of this research was that the incidence of this disease in military pets was unknown until I researched it and published it in the American Veterinary Medical Journal. These kinds of activities kept my "mankind perspective" satisfied and also caught the attention of the administrators starting the new veterinary college at Mississippi State University.

Military life was a very structured life. I was able to stay busy but, I was also required to leave work at what was for me an early time in the day. This gave me abundant free time and allowed for much time to think and create. It was during the years in the Air Force that I began formulating my future career philosophy. I wrote herd health programs for dairy and swine production facilities with which my father in South Carolina worked. I even investigated and solved some problems for him and his clients while on military leave. The free time in the Air Force also gave me the opportunity to socialize and allowed me to meet my wife. Shelley was an Air Force nurse, beautiful inside and out. Dad was to be the best man in the upcoming wedding as soon as I departed the Air Force. The dreaded conversation with my dad about veterinary practice after military service never came up. He was killed in an automobile incident the year I was to leave the Air Force. With Shelley in my life at this time, I was able to survive this crisis, and we moved to Mississippi State University in Starkville.

In due course, I realized that the work I had done through and with my dad was very satisfying, and I desired to become "an essential link in the food chain." My career philosophy became this: "If one can make an economically significant change in a food production facility, then one can stimulate the increased production of food through profits, and thereby, the world can have more to eat and possibly be at peace." This philosophy had great meaning to me because my life was significantly affected by the Vietnam War, which was originally started over food supplies. I reasoned that food supply veterinary medicine could allow me to positively affect future food supplies and peace worldwide.

My first opportunity to live into this philosophy would be to join the innovative faculty at the new Mississippi State University College of Veterinary Medicine. During my "think time" in the Air Force, I had carefully analyzed the food animal industry and concluded that if I was to create demand for my services, I needed to approach the industry from the farmer's perspective, not the veterinary school's perspective. Veterinary school typically teaches individual animal care. The farmer needs whole business care. Although the farmer enjoys producing food for others, he also desires to provide for his family while producing food. This means his farm manufacturing process needs to produce a profit like any other business. In any manufacturing process there is the necessity for sources of raw product, there is a production process which has factors that can cause losses, and there is an overall cost of production which must be managed.

In all of food animal production the source of product involves reproduction. Dairy cows must calve to produce milk, swine producers need more pigs, beef cows must calve to increase the herd, chickens need to lay more eggs, and fish must produce fingerlings for the next generation. I needed additional special training to be the best I could be at reproduction in order to increase the source of raw product. However, only increasing the source of raw product is not sufficient unto itself to create a profitable business.

There are losses during the production process in any business. In food animal production the greatest losses are due to disease. Mastitis or infection in the udder is the greatest source of loss in the dairy industry, neonatal pig disease is the most costly source of loss in swine production, respiratory disease is number one cause of loss in beef cattle, and brown blood disease is costly to catfish production. I needed to focus my veterinary education to prevent and treat production diseases.

Lastly, the greatest cost of food animal production is feeding. I needed to learn more about nutrition to better guide producers. Therefore, I set out to gain specialization in reproduction and population disease control/prevention, and I began a master's degree in animal nutrition. I completed these specialized study efforts in 1980 prepared to enter private practice and feed the world. The credentials I obtained in this specialization process set me apart (at least on paper) from most others in the field of food supply veterinary medicine and opened up many opportunities for me over the years.

CHAPTER 1
The Bomb in the Biosphere

Over the years, I realized that what drew me to food supply veterinary medicine was a passion to help mankind. My passion for feeding people and becoming a link in the food chain led me to begin collecting materials for a lecture series I eventually titled "The Bomb in the Biosphere." I began the accumulation of data when I was in veterinary school. Since this was before the internet, my sources were seminars, churches, and periodicals teaching about starvation and food shortages occurring around the globe. (Yes, there was actually serious starvation occurring during the 1960s and '70s.) I still possess original articles entitled "The Coming Famine" from 1968 and "Can Improved Production Ease Malthusian Fears?" from 1976.

Within this backdrop, just what is meant by "The Bomb in the Biosphere"? A biosphere is a round vessel containing a biological system. Our earth and its atmosphere are our biosphere containing the mass and energy interacting in such a way as to support life as we know it. The bomb is the human population explosion occurring on our earth, especially in the last century. Let me give some examples:

- From Creation until Christ, the world population was only 250 million.
- From Christ until Martin Luther in 1500 AD, the world population reached 500 million.
- During the Gold Rush of 1849, the world population finally reached one billion.
- Eighty years later during the 1929 Stock Market crash, the population reached two billion.

- Thirty years later at the inauguration of John Kennedy in 1959, the world population reached three billion.
- Fifteen years later in 1974, the world added another billion, totaling four billion.
- Thirteen years later in 1987, another billion was added, reaching five billion.
- In 1999, after only another twelve years, we reached six billion.
- Thirteen years later in 2012, another billion was added to reach seven billion.
- In 2023, the world's population now exceeds eight billion and counting (see the World Population Clock at https://www.worldometers.info/world-population/).

This is an alarming population growth explosion. Expressed in percentages, it is more dramatic. In the last half of the 20th century, the growth rate was 138 percent! The world population was growing at a rate of about 9000 per hour, or 215,000 people per day, or 78 million people per year in this era in history. The graph below demonstrates this population explosion.

World population estimates and UN projection, 10,000 BCE to 2100

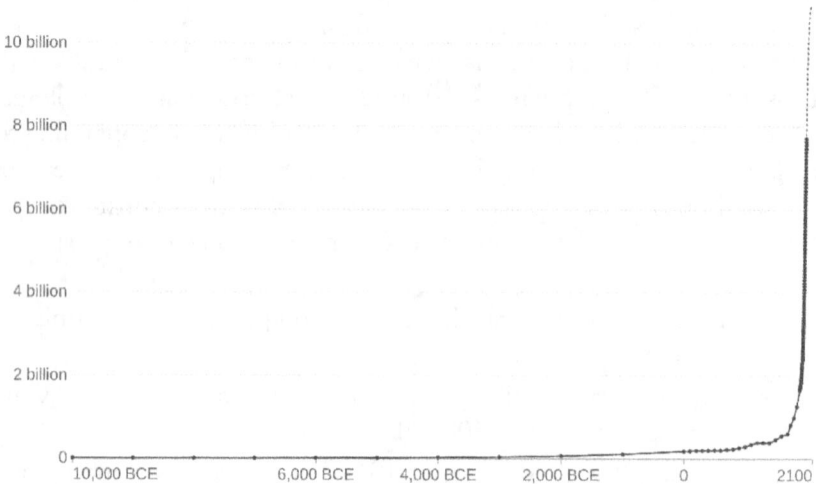

World population estimate from 10,000 BCE to 2100, by OurWorldInData, from various sources.

The starvation occurring in the 1960s and 1970s was projected to worsen by the end of the 20th century. However, it never worsened because agricultural scientists uncovered many of the secrets of plant and animal physiology and genetics. These discoveries resulted in the "green revolution" of the late 1900s. Plant physiologists determined the basic plant chemical needs, and the chemical industry developed fertilizers. Agronomy researchers began intense variety selection and hybridization of crop plants. Animal scientists researched and applied new technologies to increase the efficiency of livestock production.

An example of one of the heroes of the "green revolution" was an agronomist named Norman Borlaug, who was responsible for hybridizing wheat and demonstrating its use around the developing world. He was later credited with sustaining the lives of over three billion people. He received the Nobel Peace Prize in 1970, the Presidential Medal of Freedom in 1977, and the Congressional Gold Medal in 2006. The story of his life is inspiring to read.

So explainably, during this latter half of the 20th century, I felt "called" to help feed the world. Why did I choose veterinary medicine? I identify as a food supply veterinarian. I work with food animals, and I don't need to apologize for my work if you follow my reasoning. I chose to work with a major class of food animals called ruminants as evidenced by my degree in ruminant nutrition. Ruminants are animals with compartmented stomachs, like deer, antelopes, sheep, goats, cattle, bison, giraffes, and their relatives.

The compartmentalized forestomachs of the ruminant animal contain microbes which break down high fiber feedstuffs for use by the ruminant's true stomach, the abomasum. The "Intelligent Designer" of the universe gave ruminants to us monogastrics (simple stomached animals) because we can only utilize ten percent of the organic matter in the world, mostly seeds and roots. Ruminants can eat 90 percent of the organic matter in the world, and they are our link to the 80 percent we can't access.

Because humans, like most monogastrics, are omnivores, they gain access to most of the foodstuffs in creation through consuming ruminants or their products, such as dairy foods. In the later part of the 1900s, astounding gains in food productivity were made in animal agriculture that are comparable to the "green revolution" in plants. Today, the average dairy cow produces 2.5 times the milk quantity of the 1970 dairy cow with similar inputs. I was able to contribute to this productivity increase.

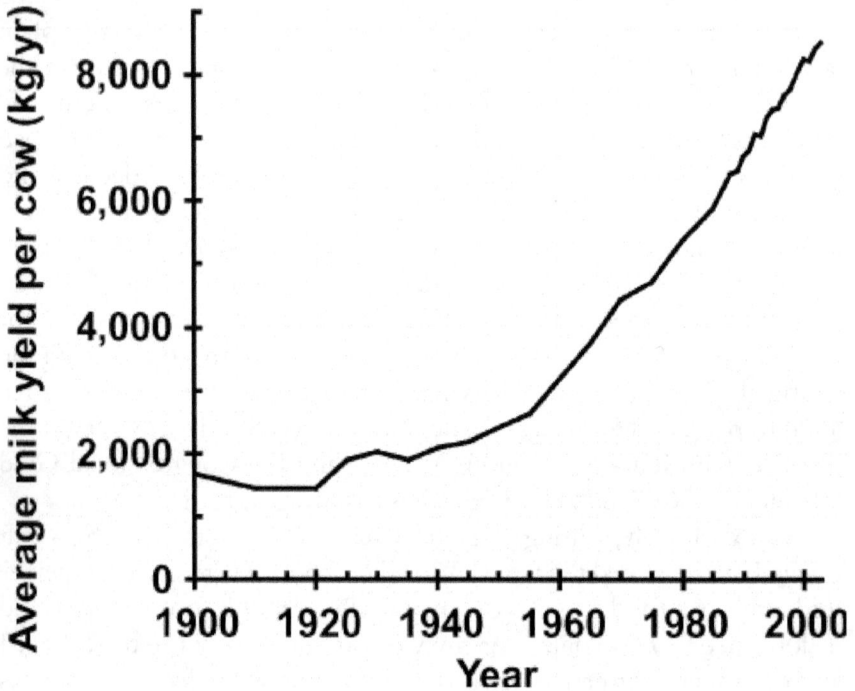

Milk production per cow in the United States over the past 100 years.
Major Advances in Nutrition: Relevance to the Sustainability of the Dairy Industry -
Scientific Figure on ResearchGate. Available from:
https://www.researchgate.net/figure/Milk-production-per-cow-in-the-United-States-over-
the-past-100-yr_fig1_7240585 [accessed 20 Jan, 2024]

The graph above shows that there have been dramatic changes in the dairy industry over the past 50 years. The U.S. is producing 60 percent more milk from 30 percent fewer cows than in 1967. When I graduated from veterinary college in 1975, a good average herd produced 12,000 pounds of milk per cow per year (a metric called rolling herd average). When I sold my last dairy herd in 2015, its rolling herd average was 30,000 pounds per cow. The technology I used in 2015 was not even dreamed of when I graduated from veterinary school. I was doing genetic probes on every calf born on my farm using hair samples. These genetic tests would indicate how much milk the resulting cow could produce, what the percent butterfat and protein would be in the milk, what the body type of the cow would be, how healthy I could expect the cow to be, and even what the pregnancy rate of the cow's daughters would be. I was genetically identifying the superior animals in my herd and multiplying their genetics beyond what was possible in nature. I was using drugs to super-ovulate them to produce dozens of fertilized embryos each year instead of the usual one calf per year. I was able to specify the sex of the calves and I could either implant the embryos into surrogate mother cows or freeze them for later use or sale.

I not only applied this novel technology in my own herd but also, in many other herds. Many of the embryos produced were shipped frozen around the world to other countries that needed genetic advancement in their national herds. Below is a cow I worked with for years. She was the top show Holstein in the world. Here she stands with 15 calves from the same collection procedure. Half of the calves are from one superior sire, and the other half are from a second superior sire. All are heifers through using sex-sorted semen during in vitro fertilization. How's that for sharing the best with the rest?!

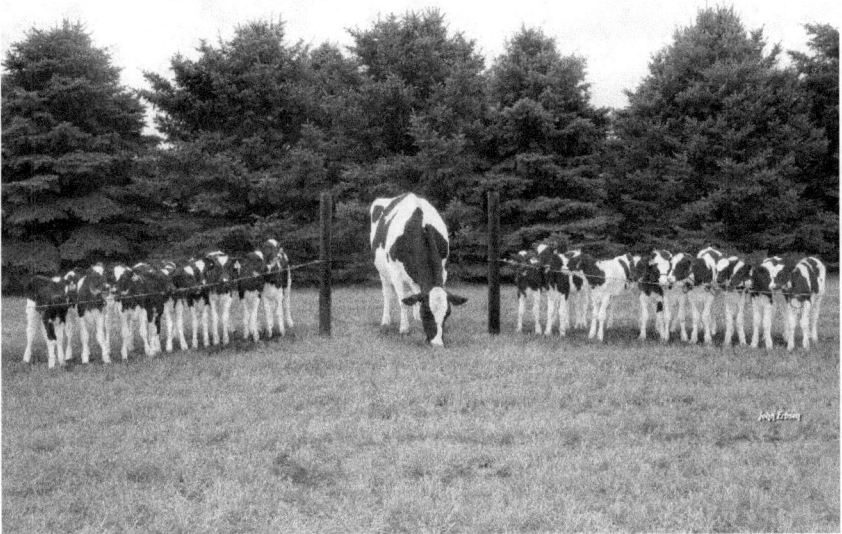

Photo credit: John Erbsen

What is more, over the years I owned four separate dairy herds, and my cows profitably produced a great quantity of food for people. Consequently, I shared the genetics and techniques I profitably used with other producers of food around the world. Much of the time, the sharing was done in developing countries while on volunteer missions. The real key to feeding people in the future will be to produce the food where it is consumed. Transportation of food from developed countries to developing countries will become cost-prohibitive in the future, if not already so.

Furthermore, as one of a few food supply veterinarians, I had the difficult task of keeping these amazing animals healthy and producing profitably while protecting the food supply. The following stories will elaborate on some of the many challenges I worked through to satisfy my passion for feeding people.

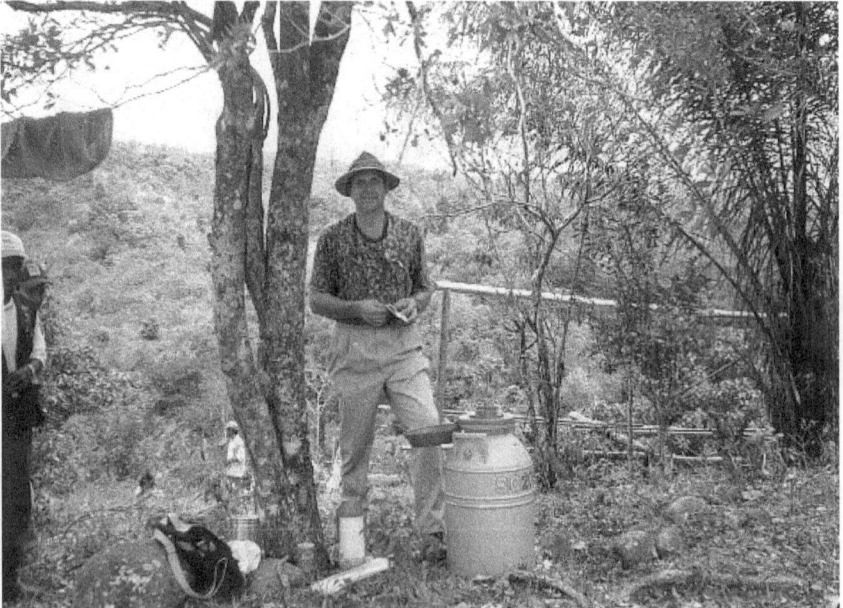

Dr. Galphin in a Bolivian jungle "lab" thawing cattle embryos for transfer while volunteering with Christian Veterinary Mission and Heifer Project International.

Although the rate of population growth has begun to slow in the beginning of the 21st century from the extreme growth of the late 20th century, it is still projected that the world will need to double food production in the next 30 years by 2050. This projection is based on current population growth statistics. The famous philosopher Yogi Berra once said, "It's tough to make predictions, especially about the future." As a consequence, the agricultural community will need to use all of the tools it can devise in order to meet the tremendous future food demand of the exploding population on our planet Earth.

This will be the great challenge for agriculture and for humanity in general—to meet the growing food demand while not degrading our environment or biosphere. The good news here is that technology is presently expanding exponentially, and it is being rapidly applied with the help of new communication tools such as the internet, digital imaging, online videos, and cell phones. Mankind has hope for a sustainable future because people are willing to fashion it. This future will be created by those who have the courage and resolve to craft it; and some of them will be food supply veterinarians.

CHAPTER 2
Environmental Benefits of Production Efficiency

All food production comes with an environmental footprint. Responsible food production works to minimize that footprint. Given how important dairy foods are to the American and the world diet, a producing dairy has a surprisingly small impact on the environment. Dairy foods provide about 16% of the protein consumed in the American diet, but the "cost" of this protein is only 1.3% of the total greenhouse gas inventory, according to the most recent Environmental Protection Agency data.

In the year 2008, the U.S. dairy industry was the first industry in the food agriculture sector to conduct a full life cycle assessment at a national level. The study showed that the dairy industry contributed just 2% of all U.S. greenhouse gas emissions. As of 2007, producing a gallon of milk used 90% less land and 65% less water with a 63% smaller carbon footprint than was the case in the year 1944.

Since 2007, thanks to increasingly modern and innovative dairy farming practices, the environmental impact of producing a gallon of milk in the year 2017 shrunk even more significantly; requiring 30% less water and 21% less land with a 19% smaller carbon footprint than it did in 2007 just 10 years earlier. This is amazing progress towards future sustainability!

Animal agriculture often gets criticized for feeding feedstuffs to animals that can be more efficiently fed directly to people. In my own dairies, I desired to demonstrate that this criticism need not be valid. I used my nutrition training to formulate rations that used no feedstuffs that competed with the human food supply. I used mainly whole plants, such as hays that are indigestible to monogastrics. I combined the whole plant forages with grain byproducts from human food processing, such as spent brewers grains from beer and hominy feed from starch production. These foods are referred to as byproducts to make the products sound desirable, but in truth, they are unwanted materials and garbage in some cases.

There was no whole corn grain, or soybean meal, or other directly human consumable foodstuff used. The cattle liked the ration and ate it well, resulting in a daily production level that yielded a 30,000-pound rolling average or an equivalent of ten gallons of milk per cow per day per year. Quite a good production level for diverting garbage from the landfill to the feed trough! It is gratifying to realize that during the 50 years of my professional life, food supply veterinarians and other agriculture scientists played an important role in feeding the global population while protecting our environment and the human food supply.

CHAPTER 3
What is Epidemiology, and What does Sherlock Holmes have to do with Veterinary Medicine?

The dictionary defines epidemiology as "the study of the distribution and determinants of health-related states or events (including disease), and the application of this study to the diagnosis and control of diseases and other health problems." An epidemiological investigation is the process of using epidemiology to find a solution to a health-related problem. When I started this book, people were not very familiar with terms like epidemiology, but after the worldwide pandemic of Coronavirus and daily briefings by human epidemiologists, everyone seems to have at least a basic understanding of this field of science.

In a population of animals, for example, one uses the powers of observation to detect what is abnormal and relate these abnormal findings to a list of possible etiologies or causes. I can still remember while in my teens, my dad stating that a veterinarian must first learn the normal before he can diagnose the abnormal. Perhaps he was trying to prepare me for my future. The distinctive skill of a successful diagnostic investigator is, therefore, the ability to probe and find the abnormal and connect the findings to a list of etiologies which are often referred to as "rule-outs" or differential diagnoses. The diagnostician then works through this list to determine the most likely suspect to be the etiology or "what done it."

Epidemiology includes diagnosis but takes the next step after diagnosis to understand the population at risk, the frequency of occurrence, the disease transmission, and the how and why. Epidemiological information is used to plan and evaluate strategies to prevent illness and as a guide to the management of patients who have already developed disease. For veterinary epidemiologists, there is also the consideration of how disease affects the food supply. The food supply must be safe, wholesome, and appealing in today's market.

I am probably not explaining the concepts involved in epidemiology very well, so as I often do to clarify a difficult concept, I will use an example. The Black Plague is a classic example of the need for epidemiology. The Plague has killed over 200 million people and countless animals over the centuries. It killed one-third of the population of Europe and as much as two-thirds of some European cities in the 14th century. It has been the most dreaded and destructive disease in history. Simply diagnosing the Black Plague became easy and routine very early in history; however, diagnosis did not change the course of the disease. This is because not enough was known about the populations at risk, the transmission, and the etiology. Epidemiology was not a thing during the fourteenth century. Germ theory was not proposed until the 16th century and was not fully accepted until the late seventeenth century after the microscope was invented. Epidemiology did not really emerge as a useful tool in health until the mid-nineteenth century.

In the fourteenth century Black Plague outbreak, doctors first thought the disease was spread by cats because they were often affected early in an outbreak. This led to the erroneous killing of cats; when actually the disease is primarily a disease of rodents, the main prey of cats. It is usually spread from rodents to other species by the flea, so when the cats were killed, the rodents multiplied unchecked and made the outbreaks worse. The outbreak in Europe was the result of infected rats being transported on ships carrying goods to ports in Italy. Then it spread to all of Europe by the movement of people and rodents.

The plague continued to periodically ravage the world for four more centuries. Epidemiologists eventually elucidated the facts about the disease, and efforts to control rodents and fleas were put in place to slow the disease. A treatment to stop deaths was actually not available until the mid-twentieth century when antibiotics were discovered. The skills of the epidemiologists greatly reduced the effects of this pandemic disease long before there was a treatment. Food supply veterinarians must possess exceptional diagnostic and epidemiologic skills when they assume responsibility for the health of food animals because they are always working with populations— herds, flocks, schools, etc.

It is difficult to develop exceptional diagnostic and epidemiologic skills. Therefore, for veterinarians, the entire last year of study is usually devoted to learning these processes in clinical rotations. I found it fascinating that the great detective Sherlock Holmes used a similar methodology in his crime-solving processes as an epidemiologist/diagnostician uses in solving health crises. He used similar skills of observation and deductive reasoning to decipher "Who could have done it." Afterward, he came up with his list of suspect "rule-outs." When I taught at veterinary college, I often told my students that I thought Sherlock Holmes should be required reading for senior students to hone their diagnostic skills. If you're familiar with the Sherlock Holmes short stories, you'll notice similarities between the process of investigation, observation, and deduction in Sherlock's stories and many of the following problem investigations that I recount in this book.

In general, maladies in animals are the result of physical trauma, infectious disease, neoplasia (cancer), metabolic dysfunction, nutritional toxicities/deficiencies, genetic alterations, or a combination of these. In addition to these major categories, there are subcategories more specific, such as virus or mineral deficiency or environmental insufficiencies. Then there are even more specific classifications, such as the specific virus or the exact mineral or toxin involved in the health problem. The following short stories will elucidate many examples of these various causes of problematic health. After the diagnosis is made and the etiology is determined, there is the epidemiology of the problem that must be deciphered to develop a problem management plan that protects the food supply.

These following stories are all based on true events, but I've taken some writer's liberties to change names and circumstances so that there is no need to obtain permission or reference scientific literature. I worked on many of the challenging cases in this book just because they were challenges. Some of the cases were accepted because the farmers and/or the animals were in need of help. Other cases were given my attention because I had empathy for the people in a community; or, because I was given a passion for feeding people. The stories and concepts in this book are intended for enjoyment, education, and provoking thought about our collective participation in preserving the future of humanity.

CHAPTER 4
CALCIUM CHAOS IN SOUTH CAROLINA

I left active duty in the United States Air Force in 1977 and began teaching at the Mississippi State University College of Veterinary in Starkville, Mississippi. This was also the year my father passed away. After his death, my mother needed help with the family farm and the livestock, so I began to drive home to South Carolina monthly to help her and manage the farm affairs. My father and I had always shared a love for agriculture and also shared the profession of veterinary medicine. These shared connections allowed me to build connections with former clients of his practice in rural South Carolina. Many of these clients I had known since my childhood as a result of visiting the farms with my father.

During one of the trips home, I was contacted by a neighbor, Mr. Weathers, who owned and operated, at that time, the largest dairy farm in South Carolina. I had visited this farm many times with my father. Weathers Farms had been experiencing increasing numbers of unusual problems in their dairy cows. The problems resulted in milk production decreases, weakness in recently calved cows, increased numbers of postpartum (after calving) diseases, and numerous down (unable to rise) cows. The problems had become very costly and were escalating, with more and more animals being affected. I had learned to appreciate the economic cost and mental stress resulting from a herd disease challenge, so I agreed to visit the dairy and investigate the problem.

The Weathers dairy was impressive. At a time when over 90% of the dairies in America were milking less than 100 cows twice a day, this farm was milking over 600 cows three times daily. The Weathers family was at the forefront of a dairy industry expansion trend that continued for decades. As a new, young veterinarian, I felt uneasy looking into a problem at a facility that had access to the best consultants in the business. Nonetheless, I began an investigation into the problem. I began examining cows for symptoms, reviewing records, observing procedures, testing inputs (feeds), and interviewing managers to initiate the epidemiological investigation into the herd's malady.

As stated previously, in epidemiology we try to elaborate a list of possible causes of a problem called rule-outs or differential diagnoses (our suspects for who done it). Examination of the cattle revealed no elevation in temperature or fever, which is a symptom of inflammation from infectious disease. This allowed me to put infectious diseases lower on my rule-out list. There was no evidence of trauma or neoplasia in live animals or on autopsy (examination of deceased animals). This left me with a metabolic cause as my most likely suspect for etiology.

The most common source of metabolic disease etiologies is the diet. Therefore I sampled the daily ration that was mixed and fed at the farm. I mailed the herd feed samples to a certified laboratory for complete analysis. While waiting for the laboratory analysis results of the feedstuffs, I gathered data on what was prescribed for feeding by the nutritional consultant working with the farm. I was able to take the nutritionist's ration ingredient recommendations and, with the aid of a computer program, perform a ration assessment that back-calculated the nutrient allowances used by the consulting nutritionist. Whenever the actual feed sample analyses were completed, I would compare the ration allowances to the actual analyses and try to determine if there were deficiencies or excesses.

Concurrently, until the feed analyses became available, time was spent calculating the monetary losses resulting from the problem. Most dairies use very elaborate computer record systems that record many important parameters such as daily milk production by cow, calving, and breeding information, and disease and treatment information. The record systems are able to analyze the data for trends and quantify them in specific time intervals. I set out to determine when the Weathers dairy began to suffer losses, how severe they were, and how long the adverse situation would be expected to go on. Some of this work would have to wait until the specific etiology was found, especially estimating when the losses would stop.

When feed reports returned from the laboratory, there was a glaring deficiency in calcium compared to the nutritional recommendations.

The suspected etiology of calcium deficiency was compared to the herd symptomatology and matched the typical signs of calcium deficiency. Adjustments were immediately made to correct the calcium levels by daily hand-addition of the calcium to the ration. This began the treatment and healing of the herd problem. Milk production slowly began to increase over the next few days, showing good response to treatment and thereby validating the diagnosis.

The next task was to find out why the calcium had been low in the first place. All feeding records were collected and analyzed for the source of low calcium. The major source of calcium in the daily cow ration was from a commercially prepared grain and mineral mix. The farm's nutritionist had specified the calcium concentration of the mix. However, the grain mix did not contain the specified calcium level, as revealed by the grain mix sample analysis. The level in the grain was only ten percent of the specified amount.

With permission from the farm, I contacted the feed company. Feed company managers found a clerical error where a decimal was accidentally misplaced when entering the feeds into a feed mixing computer. This led to the low calcium content in the finished product. The feed company admitted responsibility for the error and immediately corrected the grain mix calcium levels so the hand-feeding of calcium could stop. The feed company offered to reimburse any losses associated with the error. The process of calculating damages was made simpler by the feed company's cooperation and sharing of dates. The farmer and feed company amicably settled the calculated losses.

This early experience went so well that I gained confidence in approaching such challenging herd situations. Additionally, I realized what an important service a food supply veterinarian could provide for a farmer in trouble. Today, the Weathers family no longer has a dairy farm but one of Mr. Weathers' sons is the South Carolina Commissioner of Agriculture. Goes to show that you never know who you'll have an opportunity to meet and influence during your career.

CHAPTER 5
Milk Fever in Mississippi

While on the faculty at the Mississippi State Veterinary College, I was placed in many roles. One special role was that of Agriculture Extension Veterinarian. I functioned as a resource for county extension agents who encountered difficult livestock problems in their surveillance areas. An interesting dairy herd problem came to me from an agent in eastern Mississippi. A herd of Jersey breed dairy cows was experiencing about a 50% rate of recurring milk fever in the peripartem (near calving) cows.

Milk fever is actually the layperson's mis-terminology for a problem of blood electrolyte deficiency correctly named hypocalcaemia (low blood calcium). There is really no fever, just severe muscle weakness, usually around the time of calving when milk flow initiates. Because calcium is the major electrolyte involved in muscle contraction, low blood calcium in hypocalcemia leads to life-threatening muscle weakness. Cows go down as muscles lose the strength to support them, and if left untreated, the heart muscle will actually stop contracting, resulting in death.

Although milk fever is treatable, it must be diagnosed correctly and early. Treatment must be given immediately with dangerous intravenous calcium injections. Giving intravenous calcium too fast or incorrectly can cause cardiac arrest. The dairyman was frustrated with the number of milk fevers and was in a panic!

I felt it necessary to visit the farm with the extension agent in order to get all the facts relating to the problem. As we drove to the farm, I began my investigation by questioning him to help elaborate on the history of the problem. The herd had always experienced a small number of milk fever cases—about two to four percent of calving adult cows. This would be expected because Jerseys, as a breed, have more difficulty with calcium metabolism, and adult cows are more at risk than young females (heifers).

However, in the preceding four to five months, the cases of milk fever escalated and became more difficult to resolve. A feed company salesman had been consulted but the problem only worsened after the farmer followed his recommendations. We'll call the farmer Mr. Farmer, and he was present at the farm to give more input into the history.

Arriving at the farm, I observed a well-kept but older facility. Mr. Farmer proudly related that he had gotten pretty good at finding a cow's jugular vein and running the calcium because half of his 65 grown cows had gone down with milk fever in the past four months. He was very frustrated because, "It was just too time-consuming and nerve-racking to continue dairying in this way." He further related frustration with the feed company that told him the cause was too little calcium, so they added more to the ration. "The problem actually got worse after that change, and now almost every cow that calved was getting weak," Mr. Farmer stated. That pretty much was all he knew, so I felt the history was complete.

Next, I needed some physical facts, so I asked to see the feeding and housing areas of both the milking cows (post-calving) and dry cows (late pregnant non-lactating). While observing the dry cow situation, I found that they were allowed to graze pasture and were given a small amount of hand-fed grain. Like healthy Jersey cows, the dry cows were in good condition, alert and curious. The only remarkable finding in this group was the observation of numerous stone out-croppings in the pasture. Mr. Farmer related, "In this county of Mississippi, limestone came up to the surface everywhere and really made it hard to plow a field.

Holy Cow! There was the answer! There was no calcium deficiency, there was calcium excess! Hypocalcemia (low blood calcium) is caused by an imbalance of calcium, phosphorus, and other minerals like potassium in the peripartem (near calving) diet. Just as Mr. Farmer observed, adding calcium would make this problem worse. Hypocalcemia is not as simple as low-feed calcium.

I pulled feed samples and pasture samples to get the laboratory data necessary to verify and quantify the calcium imbalance, and I transported them back to the university lab. Within days I had the verification of my theoretical etiology. I used the lab analysis results to balance the dry cow grain mix against the pasture grass, which had excess calcium content. It was a simple fix that required decreasing calcium and increasing phosphorus. Follow-up calls over the next months to a very grateful Mr. Farmer revealed that the problem began to lessen within one week of the dry cow feed changes and had continued to improve. He thanked me for everything and then apologized boastfully for not being as easy to reach by phone as usual, "Because I've got back to fishing again."

CHAPTER 6
Arsenic on the Menu

One Friday evening, while on the faculty at Mississippi State University, I received an urgent call from a close friend named Bill McGee. He was having some problems with his calves. Bill was not only a friend, he was a mentor to me. He was a dairy science professor at the university and a committee member on my master's degree program in nutrition. Bill was also in charge of all university dairy farms and operated a very nice family dairy farm of his own.

Bill was the best cowman I've ever known, even to this day. Since animals don't talk, they rely heavily on body language to communicate. Bill could read the body language of cows with precision. I still today remember him sitting atop a large post in the cow lot, smoking his pipe and just observing the cows in their leisure activities. He was the only man who could catch one old jersey cow in heat for artificial breeding. She just looked at him in a special way when she was ready and he alone could recognize that look.

Bill was my professor in a dairy management course during my nutrition master's work that was the most informative and practical course of my degree program. He was truly gifted with "dairy sense." With this background, his calling me to help at his farm was a compliment, but it also put me in somewhat of a corner. As a faculty member at the veterinary college, I was not supposed to do local work without a local veterinarian's referral. After we discussed this complication, we decided that I was being invited to his house for lunch and I should bring my wife. I could not allow protocol to prevent me from helping a farmer friend in need. He wanted me to come visit his dairy farm the next day on Saturday, when we were both free from the classroom at the university.

The complaint he had was that his baby calves would not eat their grain and they periodically had some fresh blood in their feces. The baby calves at Bill's farm were kept in clean individual hutches or boxes and were fed milk and grain daily. Indeed, they were drinking the milk but refusing to eat much of their grain and had small amounts of blood in their feces. I examined the calves and found them to be afebrile (no fever) and very vigorous. I did observe small amounts of blood scattered in some of the manure, but the calves did not appear sick.

On questioning Bill further, I found that he had used his local veterinarian to help, and they were not able to pinpoint the source of the problem. They had done fecal cultures, which had turned out normal, and had also done a parasite screen that was negative. Nothing they did in the last week or two seemed to stop the bloody feces or encourage more consumption of the grain. Bill, in all of his experience, had never seen anything like this, and neither had his veterinarian. I continued my history gathering.

I questioned further about any other recent health problems on the farm in any animal groups. Bill, without hesitation, said the bull died that very morning. We were both unsure how this could be related, but we went to see the bull which was housed in a separate individual pen on another part of the farm. In gathering physical evidence, it was noted that the bull did not have any signs of injury or obvious concurrent disease that could have caused his death. Bill said, "He was perfectly normal the day before." The bull was housed in his own separate pen so no other animals could have caused him injury or trauma. I began to mentally make a rule-out list of things that could cause sudden death in an adult bovine. The list was not very long when you can rule out trauma and predisposing diseases. I began to focus on electrocution, toxicity, and perhaps feed bloat.

There had not been any storm the night before, and there was no electricity associated with his housing, so I removed electrocution as a cause from my mental list of "rule-outs." Feed-related problems I could narrow down through a good history, so I started questioning. I asked what the bull was fed, and Bill responded that he got a little of the same feed as the milking herd with additional access to hay, and occasionally they fed the leftover calf feed to him. I was concerned that they may have overfed the grain and caused acute bloat in the bull. But Bill insisted that they fed very little. They had severely reduced the quantity of the expensive calf feed being fed to the calves while the feed refusal problem was ongoing.

I asked who fed the calves and the bull so I could verify the quantity for myself. Bill said I could talk to his oldest son, David, when he returned from the physician's office. His son had been experiencing some vomiting and diarrhea and went in early that morning after feeding the calves to be checked out by the doctor. I moved bloat down to a lower place on my mental rule-out list.

Now I was indeed concerned, but I dared not show it. Could there be a connection between the calf problem, the bull death, and the son's health; or, were all of these unrelated? I continued my investigation by asking to see the feeds and their storage. I gathered materials to take some feed samples as I inspected the feeds. I focused on the one common feed that all had been exposed to, the calf feed. Bill pointed me toward an old abandoned concrete milk barn that was now only used for storage because he had built a newer, more modern barn.

Bill had some other chores to do and didn't think the old barn held any clues, so he left me to get his work done. I entered the old barn alone. Inside I saw three bags of calf feed standing against a large cardboard box. The bag of feed nearest the center drain in the floor was open and the only one in use. Surprisingly, there was a yellow-brown liquid running out beneath the bags of feed toward the floor drain. At first, I assumed the feed had accidentally gotten wet with water but then decided I should move the bags to find the source of the liquid. It was, oddly enough, running out of the cardboard box.

Upon opening the cardboard box I found that it contained four glass gallon jugs of an herbicide called MSMA, monosodium methyl arsenate. This is an organic arsenical or, in other words, a very toxic form of arsenic used to kill unwanted vegetation along fence rows. The farm supply company delivered both the feed and the MSMA the same day and inadvertently set the MSMA down too hard, cracking one of the glass jugs. This allowed the contents to slowly leak out and contaminate the calf feed. Wow! I needed to connect the observations I had made to deduce if the arsenic was the cause of all the problems.

Recalling the pathologic effects of oral exposure to arsenic, I remembered that it destroys small blood vessels leading to bleeding in the intestines. This could explain the blood in the calf feces. The calves apparently didn't like the taste of the arsenic-contaminated feed, and since they were getting milk, they ate very little of the feed. The bull, in contrast, seldom got grain, so he greedily consumed all he was offered. Cattle are very sensitive to arsenic, so he quickly exceeded the toxic dose resulting in his death. Bill's son, David, had handled the calf feed with his bare hands. Because this is a systemic organic arsenical, it could be absorbed through the skin.

Holy Heifer! David's illness was likely brought on by arsenic exposure. Bill and I quickly called the doctor to give him this information so that a chelating antidote could be administered to begin removing the arsenic from David's system. In this investigation, the food supply veterinarian played a role in solving animal and human illness. Happily, David experienced few problems after proper treatment and is now a grown man with a nice family of his own. As an aside, Bill passed me on the oral exams for my master's degree in nutrition.

CHAPTER 7
No Holes Bored–Wrestling with Mississippi Mastitis

Once again, in my role as Agriculture Extension Veterinarian, I received a request for help from a county extension agent, this time in a surveillance area in northern Mississippi. The agent explained that he had an experienced, successful dairyman with a recently developed, tough mastitis problem affecting his herd. To explain, mastitis (infection in the udder) is a very well-known and costly problem in the dairy world. It actually is the greatest source of economic loss in the dairy industry. I had decided to specialize in dairy farm veterinary work, so I studied everything I could find concerning this disease complex. There are volumes of material on the mastitis complex. There is even an international organization devoted to the mastitis disease complex called the National Mastitis Council. I have been a member of this organization for four or five decades.

The mastitis complex has long been recognized and referred to as the mastitis triangle because of the three main factors in its etiology (cause)—man, machine, and environment. In an effort to not turn this into a class on mastitis, I will over-simplify how mastitis occurs. A bacteria from the **environment** is forced by either a **man's** poor milking technique and/or by a malfunctioning milking **machine** through the teat orifice (where the milk comes out) up into the cow's udder, creating an infection.

The farmer named Jimmy, with the unexplained mastitis, was in real trouble. The State Department of Health monitors all raw milk shipped to milk processing plants all over the United States for food safety and quality. The Health Department had identified the changes in his farm's milk resulting from his cows' udder infections (mastitis). The farmer was about to get cut off from marketing his milk—a very costly problem that could financially kill his business.

My work was cut out for me! I would need to identify the infected cows, immediately segregate them for treatment, and exclude their milk from the market tank. I also needed to identify the bacteria responsible for the infections by culturing milk from affected cows before they received treatment. And, lastly, I needed to analyze the mastitis complex well enough to determine its root cause and correct the deficiencies, whether they be man-made, machine induced, or environmental in nature.

I traveled alone to Jimmy's farm. Alone except for all my diagnostic equipment and supplies. I was carrying a camera, a voice recorder, milk bacteria sterile culturing supplies, cleaning supplies, vacuum gauges, air flow meters, a pulsator tester (the pulsator is part of the milking system), and several milk testing kits with reagents and paddles for running a cow-side visual test called the California Mastitis Test (CMT). All of these items would be used during the day-long herd mastitis investigation. The gauges and meters would be used to check-out the milking system for proper function. Much of the machine testing would be done during the milking process to graph the machine performance with milk in the system.

The CMT kit would evaluate all of the cows before being milked so we could identify which were already infected with mastitis. The CMT detects increased numbers of white blood cells in the milk of a cow's udder responding to infection, and it allows the operator to visually assess the level of inflammation in the udder. Infected cows would have their milk sterilely sampled for later culture and identification of the causative organisms at the veterinary college microbiology laboratory. The farm environment would be observed, and the farmer's milking technique would be evaluated.

I began by observing and photographing the cows' environment. I found it exceptionally clean and recorded my findings. Next, I waited for Jimmy to bring the cows up from the pasture for milking. Before milking started, I showed him how the CMT was performed. This test was to be run on every cow so we could identify the cows already affected by mastitis. I explained that I would need his help with the CMT testing as soon as he felt comfortable running them because I needed to check out the milking system while the milking was going on. Milking time would be a busy time on this day.

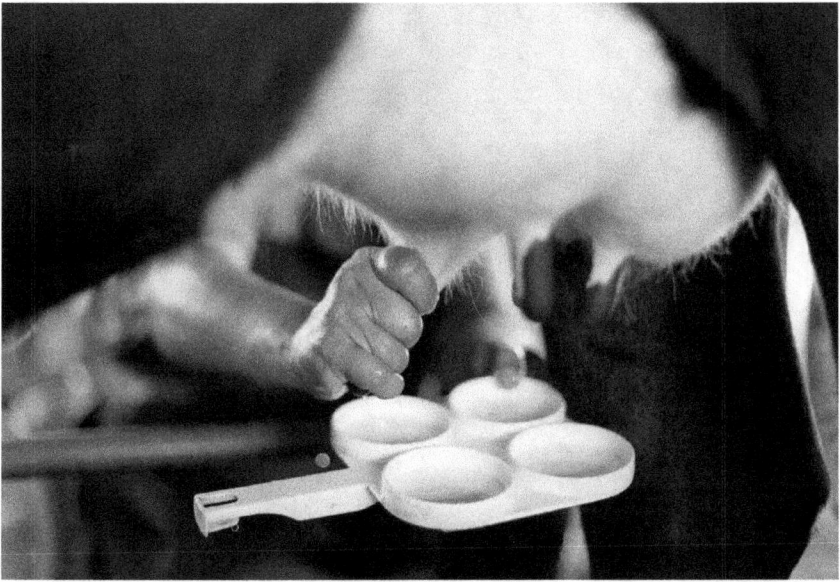

California Mastitis Test

Jimmy's milking technique was very good and should not have contributed to a herd mastitis problem.

While we worked, he told me that he felt the milking system was good because he had just bought new equipment and upgraded much of the system. The dairy equipment installer had "checked things out." I asked him if the mastitis problem was the reason for upgrading the equipment. He said, "No, but come to think of it, the mastitis started after the upgrade!" With this comment in mind I performed a thorough evaluation of the system. To my dismay, everything checked out well until I checked the last milking unit. Then "wow," there was no pulsation detectable in the last milking unit.

I disconnected the unit and inspected it. On top of the unit is a metal block where the pulsation hose attaches, and it's supposed to be bored out to split the pulsation vacuum into four small tubes going to each teat. Surprisingly, there were no holes bored in this brand-new unit to allow for pulsation airflow. The cows milked with this unit never got massaged during the milk extraction process. Every cow milked by this unit each day had their teats and teat orifices traumatized by constant vacuum, thereby setting them up for bacterial entry and infection. The fix was simple—we changed back to the old unit!

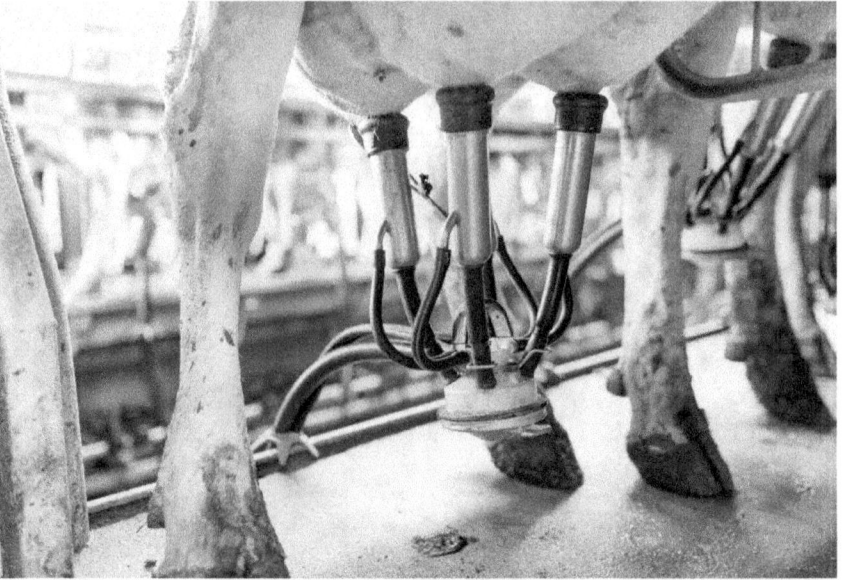

The pulsation hose is the small black hose.

Jimmy and I spoke by telephone about a week later. We had segregated the infected cows for treatment and discarding of their milk for the appropriate antibiotic clearance time. The health department had retested the herd milk and found it safe and wholesome. Jimmy's farm had been removed from the non-shipping warning list. Jimmy had not detected any new mastitis cases since the "no holes bored" milking unit was changed, and Jimmy was very happy! Later on, he and his equipment installer had a little monetary settlement discussion with the milking equipment manufacturer. The discussion must have gone well because I was never called back for an expert opinion on damages.

CHAPTER 8
Buying a Problem—Leptospirosis

It was late in the day when I received a call directly from a dairyman in east Mississippi. He got my telephone number from his son, a Virginia veterinarian. Mr. Fulper was calling about an abortion storm that had occurred in his dairy cows. He wanted some help from the veterinary school because his son lived so far away. I responded to his request and traveled to the farm the next day.

Mr. Fulper and his wife were typical early-to-rise, hardworking dairy owners. When I arrived at the farm, they were still scurrying around finishing morning chores. They took a break from work to invite me in and to help with the herd abortion investigation. They were anxious about how this problem would affect their future milk production. A dairy cow begins to increase in milk volume immediately after a normal calving and peaks in production at about 45 to 60 days in milk. After peaking, she will gradually decrease in milk volume until she calves again after another normal pregnancy.

Dairymen understand that cows produce the most milk when they are in early lactation after a normal calf delivery. It is important that a cow gets rebred as soon as possible after 60 days post-calving so that she can re-calve and resume lactating before production drops below a profitable volume. Most dairy cows have about 13 to 14-month calving intervals to yield the most profit. Abortions of calves interrupt the ongoing pregnancy and require that the cow be rebred much later in the lactation cycle, depending on the age of the fetus at the time of abortion. This delays the next calving and necessitates that the cow will have to be milked many more days while she is descending into unprofitable levels of milk production. Having too long of a calving interval is the second most costly problem in dairy herds, second only to mastitis infections. The Fulper family's anxiety was well-founded and they were ready to find and correct the cause of the herd abortion storm.

We began by recording a history of the problem. The first abortions occurred in August in five of 12 late pregnant heifers that they had purchased to increase their herd milk cow numbers. Shortly after these abortions, they had about eight of the adult dairy cows abort. The aborted calves were fairly easy to detect because they were all about four to seven months developed at the time of abortion. The fetuses were big! Their oldest son Pete, the veterinarian, came home to help them find the cows that aborted by manually palpating them for pregnancy, so there was no need to do this again. Pete did not have enough time to do anything more, and he recommended calling the vet school for help with the diagnosis. Mr. and Mrs. Fulper requested that I call Pete to let him know what was going on.

We next toured the farm to assess the condition and housing of the cows. They appeared in good health, and housing was adequate. It was noted that a pond in the lounging pasture provided both drinking water and cooling comfort for the milking cows and the late-bred heifers. The pond was fenced halfway across to keep the groups separated. I was beginning to have some suspicions about the etiology of the problem, so I asked the Fulpers to bring in the herd for blood testing. We took two blood samples from all known aborted cows and 15 percent of the other herd mates. I transported the samples back to the veterinary college and submitted them for Leptospirosis antibody testing. The excess serum was held for other tests if needed.

The veterinary college laboratory returned the screening test results for five common Leptospirosis organisms in about three days. As suspected, there were extremely high positive antibody titers to Leptospira Pomona, a common Leptospira that causes abortion storms (and there is more about Leptospirosis in Chapter 39, Lepto hardjo bovis—New/Old Problem).

The heifers purchased by the Fulpers were probably already infected when they were purchased. Mr. Fulper was irritated that he had bought the problem. After arriving at the farm, the heifers aborted and contaminated the common pond in the lounging pasture. Leptospirosis is a water-borne organism that resides in a carrier animal's kidney and reproductive tract. Some of the lactating cows drank from the pond after the heifers aborted and became infected and subsequently aborted.

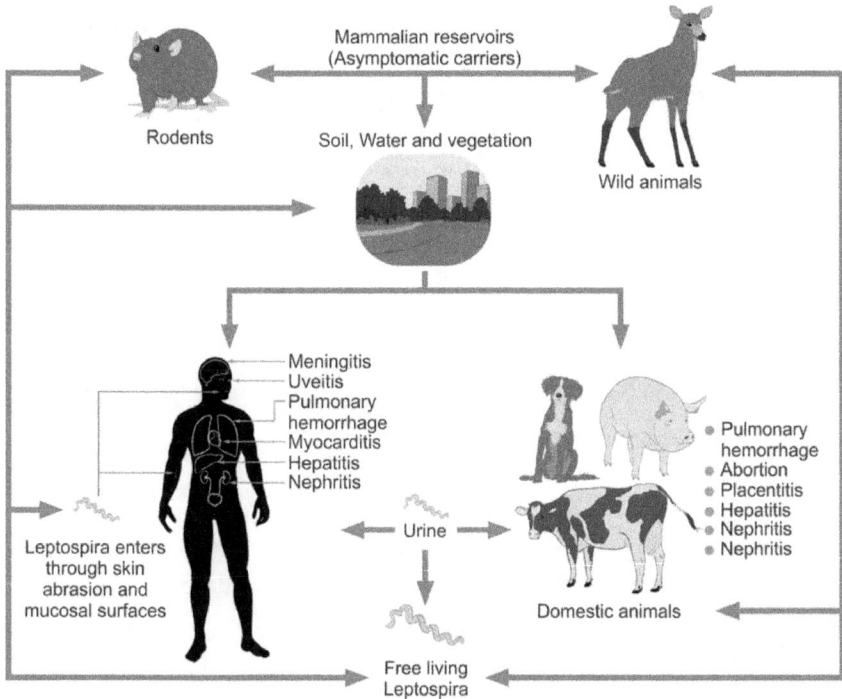

Forms of leptospirosis infection (Adapted from de Faisal et al., 2012) Rodents and other wild animals are the main reservoirs of the pathogen and generally do not develop the clinical disease. Leptospira can reach soil, water and vegetation and from there infect humans and other mammals, penetrating through damaged skin, mucous membranes and conjunctival mucosa causing the disease.

Miguel, Paulo & Meireles, Maria & Feitosa, Randyston & da Motta, Oswaldo Jesus & Pereira, Sandra & Junior, Ademir & Esmeraldo, Marcio & Montenegro, Stefania & Santana, Luiz. (2021). Leptospirosis, a clinical update regarding a neglected infectious disease. Revista de Patologia Tropical / Journal of Tropical Pathology. 49. 10.5216/rpt.v49i4.67332.

My recommendation to the dairy was to fence all cows away from the pond and provide a freshwater source from well water supplied water troughs. Additionally, they were to begin a program of quarterly Leptospirosis vaccination for all animals over three months of age for one year. Thereafter, biannual vaccination was recommended. The vaccination would augment immunity, helping to cure the infection and prevent it from spreading. The fencing of the pond would reduce exposure to the infectious organism. I cautioned them that Leptospirosis is a zoonotic disease and they should be diligent with sanitation until the problem was gone. If any of them experienced illness, they were to advise their physician of the herd problem. I related all of this to their son Pete, and they waited for his concurrence before starting on the recommendations.

During the farm visit, I enjoyed all the stories the Fulpers told about Pete, and I especially enjoyed the obvious pride they had in their son, the veterinarian. Little did I know at the time that I would move back to the Atlantic Coast in the near future and get to enjoy Pete as a trusted colleague and good friend.

CHAPTER 9
A Quick Burst of Speed Opens Doors

In 1981, I left the veterinary college in Mississippi and moved to North Carolina to join a multi-veterinarian, mixed animal, private practice in the city of Apex, North Carolina. I was given the opportunity to buy the partnership share of the senior practice partner who was leaving the business. The practice's largest client was Open Grounds Farm, a beef cattle and row crop (soybeans and corn) farm on the North Carolina coast. The farm consisted of 50 thousand acres and had five thousand head of cattle. Open Grounds measured eight miles wide by twelve miles long with one central cattle corral. The cattle never saw people on foot; always on horseback, a pickup truck, or a feed tractor.

Often when cattle were worked, a multi-mile trail drive had to be accomplished. Open Grounds Farm was a serious enterprise and the men who worked there were true professionals. All of the cattle division employees were well-trained cowboys, even up to the herd manager, who was a two-time world champion bucking bronco rider. I still, to this day, have never seen anyone who could ride and rope like this man.

When I first visited the farm, I was in awe of its size and the skills of the employees. In contrast, the farm employees were more than a little skeptical of me. To the farm personnel, I was the young vet from the city taking the place of their old, trusted, and experienced vet who was leaving the practice. I was confident in my skills; however, I knew it would take time to convince the cowboys that I was competent. The most common veterinary work performed on all the beef and dairy farms was pregnancy diagnosis.

On most farms, there was a need to know the age of the pregnancy to identify when the cow would calve again. Our practice did so much pregnancy diagnosis in dairies that we made a game of staging the

41

pregnancies accurately. We would not allow the dairyman to tell us anything. When we finished palpating (manually entering the rectum and feeling the uterus), we gave the dairyman the breeding date. It was quite amazing to the dairyman that we could pinpoint the known breeding date within one or two days. This type of diagnosis took a little more time to perform due to the need for accurate staging, but it was a good way to impress the clients.

In contrast, at this big beef farm there was no need for aging the calves because they knew when the bulls were put in and taken out of the herds. For this reason and because there were so many cattle, they were more concerned with the speed of diagnosis. They invested greatly in cattle handling facilities and expected to be able to move cattle efficiently to the corral, perform the work, and move them back to pasture on the same day.

The corral was large enough to contain two groups of 350 cows. The cowboys would move them in small groups into a central pen, called a tub. The tub was attached to a 40-foot long lane leading up to the cattle working chute that was just wide enough for one cow. The cows would therefore be lined up head to tail in the lane, ready for the individual pregnancy exams. Each herd of cows numbered about 350 head and was usually housed on a one-mile by one-mile square pasture (640 acres) some distance from the central corral. Distances often made it difficult to get two herds checked in a day.

With 5,000 breeding females on the farm, there were at least a couple of days of pregnancy work most months. Not long after I began to take over the work on the farm, they set up a two-herd day with about 700 cattle at the corral. I arrived at the farm about nine o'clock in the morning after the three-hour drive from Raleigh. The work was going along well, and in less than three hours, one herd had been completed.

During the lunch break. I noticed some discussion going on about a cow moving to the second herd. Since this was not my concern, I took time to review the pregnancy results and noted that the first herd had achieved a very respectable 91 percent pregnancy rate. After lunch, we began checking the second herd. Again, work progressed well, and after three hours, most of the herd was checked. At that juncture, there was a small break for the cowboys to consult with the manager about a cow from the first herd that was difficult to run into the tub pen leading to the cattle working chute. The cowboys suggested that she not be checked and just assumed pregnant since 90 percent had been pregnant.

At this point, I interjected that I would put the belligerent cow in the chute when I finished checking the cows standing in the lane. The cowboys countered that they had been trying to get the cow in for the entire day and had moved her into the second herd to try with that group, but had not been successful. I calmly assured them that I would try.

Open Grounds had a superb crossbreeding program based on two breeds. There were the smaller, more docile Black Angus cows and the larger, more excitable Brahman-derived Santa Gertrudis cows. This day we were working the big red Santa Gertrudis cows, and they had given the cowboys all they could handle, especially the belligerent last cow. They had nicknamed her "Ember" because she was red hot. Ember had gone into the central tub with many small groups of other cows over and over, all day long. But, before the cowboys could shut the gate to trap her, she alone would run back out all day long. Then she proceeded to run the cowboys up the corral wall all day long.

Ember determined that she was having none of this veterinarian reaching his arm up her rectum stuff. I, of course, had no knowledge of all of this anxiety-provoking activity when I hastily volunteered to put Ember into the chute by herself with no other cows around to comfort her. Methodically, I pregnancy-checked all the cows remaining in the lane as Ember watched. It was now time for me to put Ember into the chute. I removed my shoulder-length glove and strolled around to the back of the cattle lane to the location of the central tub where Ember was anxiously waiting. This was the first time I had seen her. She was a big, beautiful, tall, muscular, hyperventilating cow.

Usually, by this time of day, the cowboys were packing up or moving cows back to pasture. But to my surprise, they were all still present and sitting around the top board of the corral as if to attend a class. They weren't there for a class. They were there for a rodeo show. The pressure was on! I did not realize how badly this young city vet had insulted the cowboys when I said I'd put Ember in the chute after they had failed all day long. The herd manager tried to help me out by telling me I did not have to do this.

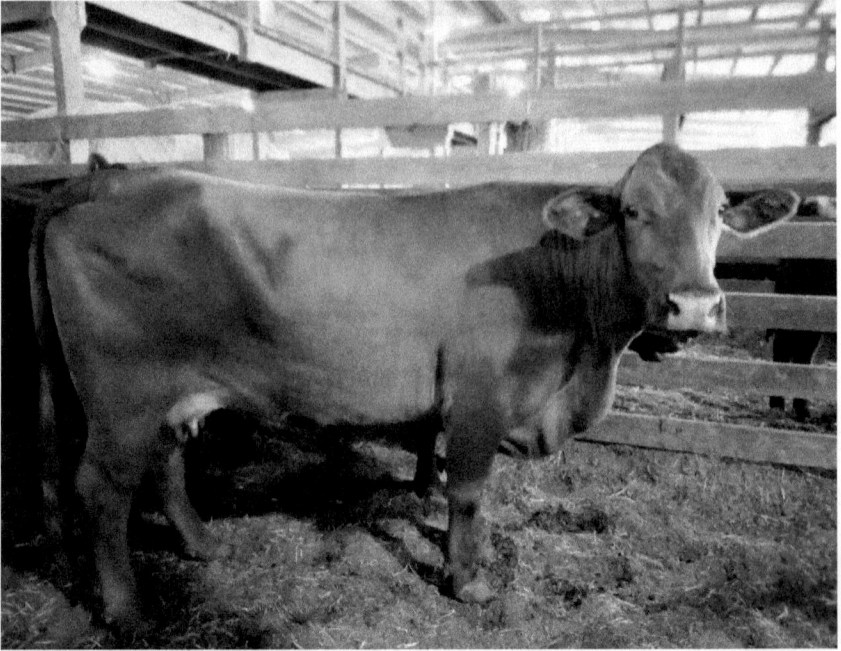

On the contrary, to save face, I had to make an attempt to get her into the chute. The cowboys typically worked the cattle with a sorting stick about the size of a finger and six feet long made of flexible fiberglass. I picked up one of these sticks and climbed down into the main corral with Ember. The corral floor was concrete, but by this time in the afternoon, was thickly covered with cow manure after 700 cows had nervously been moved over it. My rubber boots acted a little like ice skates on the slippery stuff as I approached the angry cow.

Ember was ready for this. She had practiced the chase the man up the wall" maneuver all day long. She stood with her back to the tub pen gate and faced the young veterinarian who would have to turn her around to get her into the tub. There were no other cows to distract her attention from the one man in front of her on foot and the other men sitting around the corral top, whooping and hollering like rodeo spectators.

I approached the nervous, belligerent cow and tapped the flimsy stick on the soiled corral floor about five feet in front of her. She proceeded to lunge toward me, all four feet slipping and slinging manure against the corral wall, peppering the spectators sitting on that side of the coral top. Once she got traction, she charged at me and ran me up the corral wall just as she had practiced all day long with the cowboys. The observing cowboys who had not gotten peppered with manure responded with loud shouts and clapping as if to be rooting for the cow. I regained my composure and began to lay out my next move as if I had planned what needed to happen next.

I selected four cowboys to setup along the lane between the tub and the working chute to operate stop gates. These gates would prevent Ember from backing out of the lane should I get her into the tub and up the lane. I instructed these cowboys to squat down quietly so they could not be seen as the cow went past and to then quickly shut the stop gate. All the cowboys looked at me in puzzlement as they pondered that I was just crazy enough to believe I could get that angry cow into the chute. Nevertheless, the selected cowboys complied with my instructions and took their positions by the stop gates. It was time for the rodeo finale!

I climbed down into the pen once again and approached Ember. This time, she let me get closer. I think it was because she thought she would have a better chance of getting to me before I could climb up the wall and out of her reach. I got so close that I could take the sorting stick and tap her on the nose. The tap infuriated her! Her eyes turned red hot, and she took out after me with all she had. I turned and ran in a big circle, going past her, into the tub, and down the lane. Ember was so mad that she kept coming after me with no thought of where she was going. Fortunately for me, the slippery concrete impeded her more than me. If I had fallen, she would have had her way with me for sure!

I heard the stop gates shutting behind me as I sprinted up the lane. When I got to the chute, I reached up, grabbed the top rail, and swung over the wall to safety. All the cowboys' jaws dropped, and there was silence for a second or two until they erupted into applause. I donned a new shoulder-length glove and checked Ember, finding her indeed pregnant!

This whole episode was really foolish on my part but I was young and thought I needed to overcome the assumption that I was a rookie city vet. Still, no excuse to risk my life. My skills were never questioned again at Open Grounds and whenever I made a recommendation, it was followed. That foolish quick burst of speed opened the doors to a long and successful relationship with these clients and it made a great story.

CHAPTER 10
Cotton-picking Changes

One of my favorite clients was a dairyman in Virginia named Doug Child. I felt especially close to this individual because when I arrived at the Apex, North Carolina, practice, he was not a regular client. He heard about me and our practice through other dairymen, our clients, and he was the first farmer to choose me! Initially, he called our practice for help on some individual cow emergencies. Later, he used us for emergencies, routine animal care, reproductive work, and nutrition consulting.

Doug's farm was unique. It belonged to his family since the United States was a colony, a land grant from the King of England to his ancestors. A beautiful river ran through the lower grounds, and an antebellum home stood on the highest hill overlooking the majority of the farm. The place was always well-kept, and his cows were all purebreds with the most up-to-date genetics. I enjoyed the conversations we had and the time we spent together. Doug taught me a lot, from Virginia history to cattle genetics. He also encouraged my faith journey.

At Doug's farm, the cattle were pampered and handled often, making them very gentle. At herd check time, the cows just stepped up into their free stalls and allowed me to examine them. Doug was always there to calm the cows and record my findings. During one herd visit while I was performing reproductive checks, Doug questioned me about a recent drop in milk production at his farm. Before I could respond, the cow I was examining decided to void some urine. This is just one of the unavoidable hazards of dairy reproductive work. The splashing sound then triggered cows on either side to also void. Surprisingly, the cow I was checking and the two on each side all had bloody urine.

Gee whiz! The answer to Doug's earlier question about low production was probably related to the bloody urine. A quick check around the herd revealed other cows with similar symptoms of blood in their urine. Hematuria, blood in the urine, can be caused by a number of problems. I formulated a mental "rule out" list. Trauma, cancer, infectious diseases, and toxins topped the list. Physical examination of several cows did not reveal any signs of trauma, and I was not aware of any cancer that could cause herd kidney problems. Therefore, I collected blood and urine to examine in a lab for infectious agents and possible toxins. I also pulled samples of water and feeds since all the cows had been exposed to these.

I found no elevated body temperatures or other abnormal findings that should accompany infectious diseases in any of the physical exams. Hematuria was the predominant sign, so I began to suspect a toxin that could damage the kidney. Doug was both disturbed and encouraged at the same time. He was disturbed because of the potential damage to his cows but was glad that we were quickly on a diagnostic trail towards the cause and treatment.

Over the next few days, laboratory results on blood and urine samples confirmed no usual infectious diseases were involved with the hematuria. Feed samples were clear of heavy metal toxins and farming chemicals. However, the complete mixed diet fed to the cows contained an elevated level of a mold toxin called mycotoxin T2. All the feed components in the complete mix were analyzed individually, and the analyses revealed the source of the mycotoxin was whole cottonseed. Until this instance, I had not encountered a mycotoxin problem in cottonseed. I had formulated rations for cattle for over a decade using whole cottonseed, ever since I finished my nutrition training in Mississippi where cottonseed had been plentiful. Cottonseed had always been safe because it was harvested and immediately dried at the gin before it was stored as a dry seed.

As I investigated this problem, I realized that over the intervening time period, cotton harvesting had changed as the process became more mechanized. Today, the mechanically harvested cotton containing the seed is not dried immediately but is stored in a large tightly packed bale or module and left in the field for several weeks before it is taken to the gin for drying. This cotton-picking change allowed molds time to grow on the moist seed and elaborate the dangerous mycotoxins.

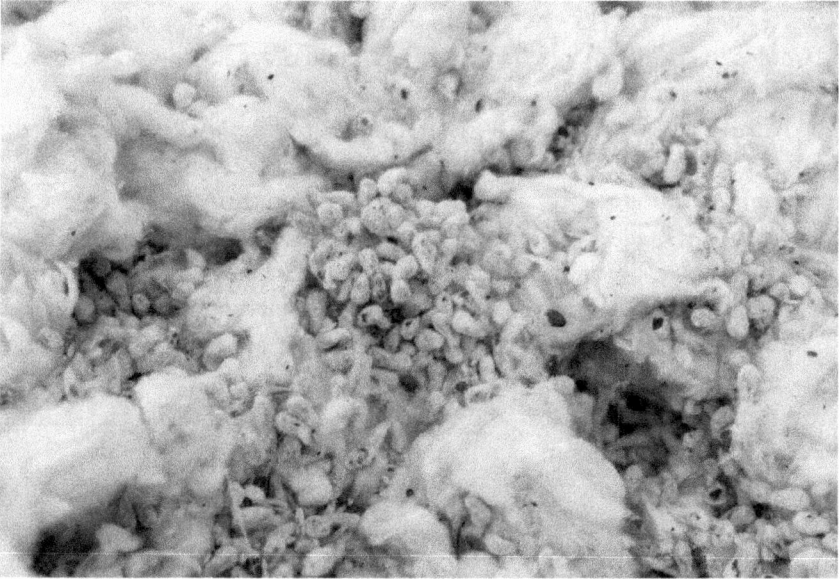

Whole Cottonseed

Doug was instructed to contact his nutritionist and immediately remove the cottonseed from the cow ration. He did this, but much damage had already been done, and he suffered substantial losses. He had to sell several cows that would not return to production, and a few cows died. Milk production suffered for many months as the remaining cows healed. Several cows aborted their calves and had to be held for rebreeding. Doug was angry and very disappointed that this had happened, as well as financially devastated. He asked me if there was a way to find out how this happened. How could a gin sell him cottonseed that was so dangerously contaminated for animal feeding purposes? I promised Doug that I would do my best to find answers and get him some help to ease his damages.

The investigation began by telephoning the gin. I informed the gin owner that there were elevated mycotoxins in seed bought from his gin and that there had been some problems. I explained that I was the attending veterinarian at a farm that had fed some of the seed. The gin owner stated that he was unaware of any problems with his seed; and besides, it was not required by state law that the seed be tested by him before it was sold. He denied any responsibility for any problems.

Such a quick, defensive answer made me suspicious that he knew more than he was sharing, so I felt compelled to investigate further. I next contacted the state university extension dairy nutritionist and

49

asked if any other dairymen had experienced problems with mycotoxins in cottonseed. I was given one dairyman's name, and I was familiar with him.

After a short conversation, I found out that he had tested the cottonseed and found high mycotoxins. He had also written a letter to the gin informing them of the mycotoxin contamination. I requested a copy and he mailed me a copy of the letter informing the gin owner. When I shared all of this information with Doug, he determined that it was time to retain a lawyer to help pursue damage recovery. Doug's lawyer determined that there was sufficient damage done and evidence of malfeasance to justify filing a lawsuit. The lawyer asked me to compile damage estimates and to be ready to act as both a fact witness and an expert witness in a civil suit.

In North Carolina and many other states, the courts are so full that one has to go through a mediation process to attempt settlement of civil suits. If mediation fails to resolve the dispute, the court system will allow you to go before a jury. Therefore, Doug and I found ourselves in a mediation. In mediation, the opposing parties do not face each other initially. They are put in different rooms, and a professional mediator appointed by the court goes between the two rooms, listening to the complaints and defenses and asking clarifying questions. The mediator does not share pertinent details with the opposing sides so as to not jeopardize later courtroom positions. He tries to point out to each side what the problems with their cases are, to encourage the opposing sides to settle out of court before taking the risk of losing all in court. Toward the end of mediation, both sides are typically brought together to work out details if there is a chance of compromise. Often, this process leads to resolutions resulting in sure settlements, albeit lower settlements.

In Doug's situation, there was no give or take by either side. The gin owner felt comfortable hiding behind the lack of state laws requiring him to test the seed before sale. He had liability insurance, and the insurance carrier was there with him, agreeing that they had no responsibility. Doug felt he could not reduce his demands since no insurance was available for damages resulting from buying a feedstuff sold as animal feed that was not fit for the intended purpose. The case seemed bound for court until I presented the copy of my dairyman friend's letter informing the gin owner that the cottonseed was contaminated with mycotoxins. The letter was dated and had informed the cotton gin owner of the high mycotoxins well before the gin sold the offending seed to Doug.

The gin insurer almost fainted when he realized the gin owner knowingly sold Doug bad seed. The insurer immediately offered to pay the entire damages claim. The insurer knew the courts had the power to triple damages if fraud could be proven. The insurance company could not take that risk. Doug only wanted to be compensated for his actual losses, so he walked out of mediation with over $100,000 to begin the healing of his dairy business. I walked out feeling that I had truly helped a friend stay in the business he loved—producing food.

CHAPTER 11
Please Pass the Salt

While attending a national continuing education seminar called The American Association of Bovine Practitioners (AABP), I overheard conversations in the hallways about a problem at the largest dairy in South Carolina. Rumor was that 20 or more of the highest-producing cows had died suddenly and that the problem had been looked at by some of the best veterinary consultants in the business. The problem was still unresolved after numerous specialists had formulated diagnostic and corrective theories that did not work.

I was concerned about this dairy business, and I was also curious as to whether the dairy could be the Weathers family farm. They were the friends I had helped with my father when visiting my home from Mississippi. At that earlier time Weathers Farms, Inc. had been the largest dairy in South Carolina. So, after leaving the AABP convention and returning to my home office in North Carolina, I made a telephone call to Weathers Farms, Inc.

Mr. Weathers answered the phone with an anxious tone. He related that they had been struggling with multiple death losses in his highest-producing cows. He had called every dairy specialist and veterinarian he could think of but had not remembered me. Last he knew, I was still in Mississippi teaching at the vet school. My father had passed away, and other veterinarians were now doing his veterinary work. He said he was sure glad I called because nothing was getting any better. He knew I lived far away but hoped I could find a way to come there for a visit.

I liked Mr. Weathers because he always spoke what was on his mind. He invited me to his dairy to have a turn at trying to solve this problem. I made immediate plans for a trip to his farm which was only 15 miles from my family's farm and my mother's house. Ironically, I actually had been traveling to this area from North Carolina every month since my father's death, in order to visit my mother and help her with our family farm. Making a visit to Weathers Farms, Inc. would only make my home visit more productive.

Mr. Weathers and his sons met me when I arrived. The sons were now doing most of the day-to-day management as Dad Weathers transitioned to retirement—a necessary process on most family farms. The older son was managing the crop farming enterprises, and the younger son was managing the dairy enterprise. I was assigned to the younger son for my briefing on the ongoing death loss problem. The farm was milking 700 cows. Death losses numbered 23 to 24 adult cows, all from the two high-producing groups, which numbered 85 cows each.

The affected cows were just randomly found dead in the housing area between the twice-daily milkings. This was an astounding 15 percent of the high-milking groups dying suddenly at random times! Autopsies had been performed on many of the deceased cows, but nothing remarkable had shown up at the state diagnostic laboratory. This fact was notable to me because whatever was killing the animals did not have time to damage any organ systems.

A consulting veterinarian who worked with them first proposed that the problem could be Black's disease, a bacterial infection with sudden death and very few symptoms. He had the farm vaccinate all the cows twice for Black's disease, but the death losses continued. Secondly, the consultant suggested that the new crop of whole cottonseed in the ration contained a toxin. The farm had started feeding it just prior to the initial deaths. The cows had increased consumption of sodium bicarbonate mineral, considered to be a digestive system protectant by the consultant, in the same time period. The farm stopped feeding the cottonseed and tested it for toxins, but it tested negative. The consultant surmised that the offending seed had already been fed up, but the deaths had continued after removing the cottonseed. No theory or plan of action had achieved any results, and the death losses were expensively, frustratingly piling up.

Seven years passed since I had last been on this farm. It was still the largest dairy in South Carolina, and the facilities occupied the same footprint. But the feeding system had been modernized. On my initial visit to the dairy, they were feeding forages in outside troughs and feeding a purchased grain mix in the milk barn while milking. Now they were feeding a free choice (ad libitum) total mixed ration with grains and forages precisely blended in outside housing area feed troughs. This new feeding technique gave the cows more time to eat and prevented the digestive upsets caused by twice daily slug feeding of large amounts of grain in the milk barn while being milked.

The new total mixed ration (TMR) technology was the feeding method I preferred, and I had been busy converting my clients in North Carolina to TMRs for the preceding five years. TMRs had other advantages besides fewer digestive upsets, such as lower feeding costs. They importantly allowed a farmer to feed less expensive, directly purchased byproducts and feed commodities that bypass the feed company price markups. However, the farmer had to acquire the skills to purchase, handle, store, weigh, and properly mix the ration on the farm. TMRs also required the services of a nutrition consultant to formulate a proper ration that includes not only the macro elements like protein, energy, and fiber but also all the minor ingredients like minerals and vitamins.

I knew from my previous work with Mr. Weathers that the farm kept meticulous, detailed records. With the oral history-taking and feeding management changes as a base of knowledge, I was ready to delve into the records. The autopsy reports were just as described with nothing to discover, but I did note the time that the death losses began. I visually observed the two high-milking cattle groups finding nothing out of the ordinary. I looked at the milk shipment records and the milk quality data finding nothing remarkable. Then I examined the feeding program records to see when the increased consumption of sodium bicarbonate (bicarb) began.

The bicarb was being fed only to the high milking groups as a free choice (ad libitum) mineral in a wooden mineral box outside in the housing area. Interestingly, bicarb consumption went from zero to a quarter of a pound per cow per day the week before deaths began. Then the week that the first deaths occurred, the bicarb consumption jumped to over three pounds per cow per day. At the time of my visit, the farm was having difficulty finding enough bicarb to buy because the groups were eating over two tons per week and had been doing so for several weeks. I had never seen a cow voluntarily eat over a quarter pound of bicarb per day, so I was sure the deaths were somehow related to this high bicarb consumption. I needed time at my computer to analyze the current ration, so I made a copy of their feeding program for later analysis, knowing I would return to the farm the following day.

Overnight I looked at the ration and compared it to what I would have done. Everything looked good, except there was no salt (sodium chloride) in the ration. I was always careful to put at least one-tenth of a pound of salt per cow per day into my mixed rations because my training taught me that salt is a daily required nutrient. Often farmers put out free choice saltboxes, but if the boxes were to accidentally get empty, I always had salt inside my complete mix.

Armed with this ration analysis, I returned to Weathers Farm the next day to get answers to the question, "Where's the salt?" The answer was, "There's no salt!" I had found a major problem, but I was puzzled about how this could have happened and how it was causing the deaths.

The current nutrition consultant relied on the farm to put salt outside in mineral boxes. This had worked well until the farm management contacted another nutrition consultant looking for a way to "tweak" the high group ration to get more milk production. The second nutrition consultant suggested feeding free choice bicarb as a way to get more feed consumption and thereby higher milk production. Farm management did not share this suggested change with the current nutrition consultant but instead went ahead and put bicarb in the mineral boxes in the place of the salt. Thus, the high-milking groups had no salt. Farm records of salt and sodium bicarbonate purchases verified the changes and identified the date cow deaths began.

When cows are salt deprived they develop a condition called "pica" which is the tendency to eat abnormal things. The high-producing cows consumed the bicarb in large quantities trying to satisfy their salt craving. Actually, the procedure on the farm was for the mineral boxes to be filled while the cows were in the milking barn. Therefore, the first few cows that were turned out of the barn after milking probably ate all of the bicarb in the boxes. Sodium bicarbonate is a powerful buffer that lowers the acid measure of fluids called the "pH." If a cow could quickly eat enough bicarb, it would cause a drop in stomach pH and in turn cause a drop in blood pH, which would be fatal. The pica could lead to a fatal "metabolic alkalosis."

The immediate fix I came up with that day was to split the mineral box in half by installing a divider board. Salt was placed on one side and bicarb on the other side. I knew we had solved the puzzle the very next day when bicarb consumption in the high groups decreased to a quarter pound per cow per day. With the decrease in bicarb consumption, the death losses immediately stopped. The high milking groups soon began consuming the normal 10 to 15 hundredths of a pound of salt per head per day. My reward for the detective work was a new old client. I worked with the Weathers family dairy for decades after that until they exited the dairy business. And the cows said, "Please pass the salt!"

CHAPTER 12
HOUR PLACE FARM IS MISNOMER

The first dairy business I actually had ownership in was legally named Hour Place Farm. I shared the ownership of this business with my friend and veterinary partner, Dr. Ben Shelton. Dr. Ben and I both did cattle veterinary practice at our hospital and shared a love of dairy cattle and the dairy business. We had often dreamed of owning some cattle of our own. It seemed natural for us to take advantage of one of our best client's offer to sell us his cows and to begin a dairy business of our own together. The client was also willing to rent us his farm and facilities. He was getting older and wished to retire from the 365 days a year work schedule he had endured his entire adult life.

Dr. Ben and I could not have financially afforded to get into such a business without his agreement to personally finance our purchase of his cows and to rent us his farm. We were naively sure the cows would milk enough to pay for themselves and pay the rent under our smart management. We were more than a little naïve when we named the business Hour Place Farm, thinking we would spend only an hour per day checking on things and managing our hired help.

Except for that assumption of only an hour of work per day, things were going along pretty well at the farm for the first couple of years of our seven-year contract. Then one afternoon Dr. Ben noticed that the milk production had dropped drastically. He called me in for another hour or so of work while we investigated the sudden milk production drop. We observed all of the cows and the milking process to detect any health problems but found nothing wrong there. We reviewed the feeding program and examined the recently delivered feeds but found nothing unusual. A plan was made for me to return the next day and spend the entire day at the farm. I went home and called the clients scheduled for herd calls the next day and canceled the herd visits. I had never canceled a day's work before!

Early the following day I arrived at Hour Place Farm with a checklist of investigative tasks. I helped with the feeding and milking. Nothing appeared to be out of order. The cows ate the feed and milked out cleanly. I checked the scales on the feed weigh boxes and on the feed mixer wagon. Everything checked out to acceptable tolerances. Eventually, I went into the milk tank room and checked the volume of milk in the milk storage tank. Production was still depressed. However, while in the tank room, I noticed the milking system wash vat didn't completely fill with water before the wash cycle started. I wondered who had messed with the timer because I had properly set up the wash system myself a month earlier. I next used an electronic meter to scan the premises for stray electric voltage.

I had found stray voltage in several old barns like ours over the past years. Stray voltage interfered with milk letdown and caused cows to produce less milk. No stray voltage was detected. The last check I had on my list was to perform an evaluation of the milking system function. Vacuum levels were holding steady at the proper setting of fourteen inches of mercury, and pulsator function was normal. Lastly, I went outside to check the vacuum pump for airflow and found the required ten cubic feet per minute of airflow for each milking unit. Everything in the milking system checked out to be properly functioning. I had not yet found a cause for the sudden decrease in milk production.

While outside reassembling the vacuum system I stood up to scratch my head over the puzzling dilemma of the low milk production and I noticed a couple of cows fighting beside a little automatic water trough. At that point, a third cow came up and shoved the other two and a fourth cow came over and joined the skirmish. This was definitely unusual behavior for my sweet cows! I walked over to the waterer and found it empty and the water flow was very slow. Remembering the failure of the wash-up system vat to fill before the cycle started, I quickly realized I had a water pressure problem. This served as a good lesson that not all rapid milk production drops are the result of disease, incorrect feeding, equipment malfunction, or nervousness.

Milk is roughly 90 percent water, and if you interfere with the milk cow's water consumption, production will rapidly decrease. This was a cooler time of year, so there was not an excessive need for water, and there was no voltage detected preventing consumption, and the water was fresh from a well, so it was not tainted. Therefore, there must simply have been a shortage of supply. It was time to check the wells and water system.

We were fortunate to have two wells and two pumps supplying the farm water. I first looked in the main pump house on the milk barn's east side. The pressure gauge on the water holding tank registered the proper pressure level of 60 pounds per square inch, and everything else appeared normal. I then checked the backup water pump located on the west side of the milk barn in a small building we used as a farm office.

There I found that the valve connecting this pump to the milk barn had been turned off. It was usually turned on. We had over 250 total animals on the premises, counting all of the young stock. I surmised that the main pump could not supply enough water by itself for all these animals and the backup pump was needed. So I turned the valve back open. I walked back to the previously slow-running water trough and found it filling fast, and cows were no longer waiting in line for water. I left the farm feeling satisfied that the problem was resolved. The next day Dr. Ben telephoned me to tell me that milk production had returned to normal.

Nonetheless, four days later the milk production dropped again. This time I looked straightaway at the water supply and found the backup well valve turned off again. Since we were renters, I marched over to the landowner's house to query him about the dilemma of the closed valve. He told me that he had closed the valve because that well had failed and he had to replace the pump at considerable expense. That well supplied his family's home, and he preferred to keep it isolated for the home to reduce the load on the well pump. He assured me that the main well had always supplied enough water for the cattle in the past. Nevertheless, he agreed to allow me to join the two wells until I could find the solution to the main well's supply shortfall. As a renter, my only recourse was to thank him for allowing us the time to correct the problem because one doesn't want a bad relationship with the landlord.

I called well specialists to the farm to pull up the pump and lines to the water tank. They were unable to find any problem and could not explain the slowness of the water flow, since the tank pressure and supply were normal. The specialists left the farm still baffled. I, myself, began taking pipes apart from the holding tank to the barn and after much effort finally found the source of the slow water supply. The steel holding tank was linked to the steel barn water pipe by a plastic hose clamped onto a cast-iron hose fitting. The cast-iron hose fitting was stopped up by iron deposits, closing it so tightly that a wooden pencil could not get through. Imagine trying to water 250 large animals through a pencil-sized opening—not possible. Because of the differences in metals in the supply line (cast iron and steel), an electrolysis process was set up that electrolytically welded the iron in the water to the surfaces of the iron fitting. I replaced the damaged fitting with a new one-inch diameter fitting and resolved the slow water dilemma.

Hour Place Farm became an award-winning, profitable investment, and Dr. Ben and I received valuable on-the-job training almost daily. It made both of us wiser dairy veterinary consultants. After a few years, we branched out even further setting up Hour Place II simultaneously with Hour Place. Eventually, we developed a dairy cow sharecropping business we named G&S Cattle for Galphin and Shelton. This business shared dairy cows with our clients who needed additional animals to help increase their cash flow and enable debt service. G&S Cattle had about one thousand cattle scattered in herds across the southeastern states. We helped many clients avoid bankruptcy and even helped some clients out of bankruptcy.

Dr. Ben and I also benefited in another less tangible way. By being owner-operators of successful dairy businesses, our clients attributed more legitimacy to our recommendations. This greatly increased demand for our food supply veterinary services. At the end of our contract at Hour Place Farm, emboldened by our successes, both of us created new opportunities for ourselves. Dr. Ben bought his own dairy farm in western North Carolina using Hour Place cattle as a starting herd. He also operated his own veterinary practice from his farm location. I went on pursuing my passion for feeding people by continuing my stateside food supply veterinary practice, S Galphin Services, by starting an international dairy consulting company, Worldwide Agriculture Consulting (WAC), and by owning two additional dairy farms under the name of Agri-Science Opportunities, Inc.

I have a close friend who was a young county extension agent when we first met. He asked me if I knew anyone at the state agriculture college in Raleigh who could help him with an advancement opportunity. I replied that a man of his training should create his own opportunities. At the time this was not what he wanted to hear and he became angry with me. A few years later when we were working together again he apologized for his initial reaction to my advice. He told me that after thinking about it he realized it was the best advice anyone could have given him. He followed the advice and created his own opportunities as he rose to director of the whole county extension service. The Hour Place Farm experience taught Dr. Ben and I to never stop learning and to create our own opportunities. I pass this same advice on to you readers: never stop learning and create your own opportunities.

CHAPTER 13
Farming Is a Dangerous Business

As mentioned in an earlier part of this book, reproduction is the source of income in food animal agriculture. Dairy cows must calve every 12 to 14 months to produce maximum amounts of milk. Beef cows should calve yearly to have calves for sale and replacement females. Hogs need to have more pigs per litter and more litters per year to make a swine business profitable. And so on, this applies to all of the other food animal industry groups.

For this reason, a food supply veterinarian spends much time doing reproductive work. For years, most of my time was spent doing routine reproductive checks on cows that had been bred by my clients artificially or by a bull. My role was to identify which cows did not become pregnant to a recent breeding so that the cows could be put in a program for rebreeding. I visited most of my dairy clients at least monthly to check their eligible cows for pregnancy. The regular, repetitive nature of this work had the benefit of me getting to know my clients very well. This story is not about animals but the client farmers and the dangers they face in their work.

It was early afternoon, and I was headed to my next appointment to check pregnancies at a small dairy near Buies Creek. The location of the dairy was a beautiful, flat area in central North Carolina just north of the Cape Fear River in the fertile river floodplain. The farm was owned by two elder brothers but most of the work was done by their adult sons David and Tye. Tye was the cowman at the farm and enjoyed working with the animals. He was always present for the routine pregnancy checks. Tye was a very motivated and punctual person, so as a result, everything was always ready when I arrived for herd work.

This day was different. I saw all the milk cows still grazing outside in the pasture as I left the highway and turned onto the farm path. I suspected that something was awry. Tye's truck was parked in front of the barn, but Tye was not there leaning on it and waiting for me as usual.

I wandered around the barn to find someone. After looking in the feeding area and the milking parlor I finally found Tye in the office with his head down on the desk. He was very still and very pale, but he raised his head as I entered the small room. He began to apologize for not being ready and stumbled as he tried to rise. I steadied him, helped him return to the desk chair, and then began to ask questions. He told me he felt fine when he came to the barn early that morning, but over the last six hours, he had begun to feel nauseous and experienced some vomiting and diarrhea. He had gotten a little dizzy and came into the office to recover some time ago, but he was not sure how long he had been resting.

His physical/clinical signs concerned me so I asked what he had done that morning. He said he had sprayed a weevil control chemical on the alfalfa field after feeding the cows. I asked what product he used, and he responded "Furadan." I next enquired if he had spilled any of it on himself, and he acknowledged that he had spilled some of the concentrate on his jeans when he was mixing it. He was still wearing the jeans! My knowledge of this dangerous carbamate pesticide told me that this could be a serious problem. I had experienced a herd toxicosis before, when cattle were allowed too early access to recently treated areas. I asked where the product was located so I could examine the label. I attach portions of the label here:

> *User Safety Recommendations: Users should wash hands before eating, drinking, chewing gum, using tobacco or using the toilet. Remove clothing immediately if pesticide gets inside. Then wash thoroughly and put on clean clothing. Remove personal protective equipment (PPE) immediately after handling this product. Wash outside of gloves before removing. As soon as possible, wash thoroughly and change into clean clothing.*

Another part of the label read,

> *If on Skin or Clothing: Take off contaminated clothing. Rinse skin immediately with plenty of water for 15·20 minutes. Call a poison control center or doctor for treatment advice. Contains*

an N~methyl carbamate that inhibits cholinesterase. Have the product container or label with you when calling a poison control center or doctor, or going for treatment. You may also contact 1-800-331-3148 for emergency medical treatment information.

With this information, we quickly removed his soiled clothes and thoroughly washed his legs and hands with soap and water. Afterward, we called his local physician, and I sent him to the doctor with a clean copy of the label. I shudder to think that had it not been for the scheduled pregnancy check, Tye may have laid there on his office desk too long to overcome the effects of the Furadan. As it was, adequate efforts were made in a timely manner, and the incident led to no eventual harm. Unfortunately, this is not always the case for all pesticide-exposed farmers. The need to use these types of dangerous products makes farming a dangerous business!

CHAPTER 14
En "Counter" with Death

The telephone startled me awake from my bed at home in Raleigh at four o'clock in the morning. I worked my turn on emergency calls for the veterinary practice, but I wasn't on emergency duty that night or morning. On the phone was my friend and client Joe and he was frantically trying to give me the details about something terrible happening at his dairy. When he arrived at the barn to milk that morning, he found three cows dead and four more down.

"Could you come right away?" He asked.

"Of course I will. Let me get dressed, and I'll leave right away," I responded.

Joe's farm was about an hour away. I had great respect for this farmer. He was able to successfully dairy with only one normal leg. He had lost one leg in a farm accident but had not let it stop him from doing what he loved to do—dairy. He was a little older than many of our other clients because he had served in the army during the Korean conflict before he returned home to start his dairy. Because he had more life experience, Joe always seemed quiet, patient, and humble in his demeanor. The panic in his voice on that early morning telephone call distressed me.

It was still dark when I arrived at Joe's farm, and to my surprise, there were now six dead cows with several more down. This truly was a catastrophe in the making! I began examining the live cows hoping to find some clues. The live down cows had no elevated temperatures. They were very depressed and had little to no internal gut sounds. Most were drooling saliva, and their heart rate was slow to irregular. There were moderate signs of diarrhea, and urine appeared normal. The pupils appeared to be tightly closed (meiotic), and muscles were fasciculating or contracting irregularly. These signs resembled an acute toxicosis of some kind.

But what toxin? Was it in the water? Was it in the feed? Which one of the feedstuffs? Are all groups on the farm exposed? What kind of toxin was so powerful it could kill and sicken so many adult cows, each averaging 1,500 pounds in body weight?

Joe's brother was available to drive one of the most recently deceased cows to the diagnostic lab in Raleigh, about 60 miles away. He could get there as they opened if he left immediately, so we loaded a cow on a trailer as the first task. I then gathered samples of the water, the individual feeds, and the mixed feed from the holding area. I also took a sample of the milk they were harvesting so we could determine if it was safe to sell.

It would be several hours before we could hear results from the diagnostic lab. I had a little work to do at a nearby farm so while we waited on the lab results, I slipped off to do the previously scheduled work. I instructed Joe to shut the cows away from the feed bunk and water while I was gone. We would resume the investigation when I returned in about three hours. While on the road to the neighboring farm, I telephoned the lab to notify them and give them my history and clinical findings from the cow physical exams. I didn't know what toxic agent to have them test for because Joe insisted that he couldn't think of anything toxic on the farm.

I returned to Joe's farm earlier than predicted—it was only eleven o'clock. In just that short time, there were five more dead cows and seven additional down cows. The diagnostic lab had insufficient time to get any results, so Joe and I began to walk about his farm to see what we could discover. We went into the empty holding lot where the feed bunk was located, and I noticed that the bunk was empty. I fearfully asked Joe if he had let the cows back in to clean the trough, and he said he had removed the feed and told the feed truck driver to dump it on a concrete floor until later. I walked over to the feed bunk to verify that all the feed was removed and was stunned to find several dead and dying mice in the trough. The dead mice "told" me that the toxin was in the mixed feed in sufficient amounts to kill the mice.

I immediately telephoned the lab to inform them of the toxin source. Joe and I continued our walkabout with emphasis on where and how the feed was mixed. The minerals and vitamins for the milk cow ration were added to the mix near an old shelter across the highway from the milk barn. While reviewing the mixing procedure, I asked Joe if there was anything toxic in the adjacent old shelter. He said there was a pesticide called "Counter" in the barn which was used on corn seed at planting, but the barn stayed locked at all times, and he had the only key. He was sure no one could get to it.

I continued to look around and noticed the machinery shed was nearby with the corn planters parked underneath. I walked over to the planter and opened the pesticide hopper to find the toxic substance half-filling the hopper. The toxic "Counter" was not all locked up! I immediately telephoned the diagnostic lab with the name of my suspected toxin, the powerful organophosphate pesticide Terbufos, trade named "Counter." An hour later the lab telephoned with positive results for "Counter" in the feed and in the autopsied cow.

We had determined our toxin and source of exposure, and now we needed a treatment plan to manage the problem. Finally, we needed to determine how the toxin got into the mixed feed in the first place. The best available treatment at the time for organophosphate poisoning was a drug called atropine which is not an antidote but is capable of reversing a few of the symptoms. An oral drench called activated charcoal was also recommended to chelate or bind some of the toxin in the gut. I had a few doses of both of these compounds on my veterinary truck so Joe and I began administering what I had to some down cows.

It was at this time that one of Joe's men came up and said that some heifers in another group were showing similar signs to the cows. We finished treating cows with the few doses I had with me and we went out to the affected heifer group. Sure enough, the heifers were displaying symptoms of organophosphate toxicity also. Joe did some questioning and found out that the feed truck driver had misunderstood his directions that morning, and he had remixed the contaminated feed with additional corn forage and delivered it to the pregnant heifer group. We calculated that there were at least 150 grown cows and heifers exposed to the poison.

This changed the dynamics for obtaining drugs for treatment. We would potentially need enough material to treat 150 large animals. I telephoned my clinic and asked that the staff start locating all available atropine and activated charcoal in eastern North Carolina. Joe and I talked further about how the toxin could have gotten into the milk cow feed. He had no idea unless a disgruntled former employee could have come at night and thrown a handful of "Counter" into the feed wagon, which would have been pre-filled for the early morning feeding. As a temporary fix to prevent anything like this from happening again, I suggested that the feed be mixed immediately before delivery to the feed trough by a trusted employee. Joe agreed!

It was late afternoon, so I told Joe that I needed to return to my clinic and begin the process of gathering treatment materials. I would return the next day as early as possible to deliver the drugs and help with treatments. I spent the evening driving to pharmacies to pick up atropine and activated charcoal. I also rescheduled my work for the next day so that I could devote all my time to helping Joe.

When I arrived at Joe's the next morning the scene looked like a battlefield. There were in excess of 30 dead cows scattered around the cow pasture. Another 15 or so were down. Joe had hired an excavator to dig a large trench on the far side of the pasture to dispose of the dead. He was busily dragging the dead bodies to the trench. I got him to pause this depressing activity and help me for a while as we treated all of the down cows with atropine and charcoal. It took hours to orally drench so many cows, but the act of treating the cows was therapeutic for both Joe and me. We felt some hope that we could reverse some of the damage done by the toxin.

At noon that day, we took a short break and then resumed the removal of dead cows to the burial trench. All afternoon that day we took a tractor, hooked a chain to the dead, and dragged the animals across the pasture to the trench. Many of the animals we had treated were also dragged away as the treatments failed to stop the dying. By nightfall, Joe and I realized we would just have to wait and see how many of the cows had eaten enough of the contaminated feed to kill them. Our treatments were doing little to change the outcome.

The next day we continued the treatments until the drugs were all used up. We then resumed removing the dead to the trench. By early afternoon we had caught up with the burials. Joe and I sat together under the shade of the barn and assessed the situation. Of the 130 milking cows and 25 pregnant heifers, we had saved only 45. He now only had 35 cows to milk and some of them were weakened by the toxin. He was essentially out of business!

With wet eyes, I asked, "What will you do now, Joe?"

He answered, "I don't know how to do anything but dairy. I don't want to do anything else. I guess I'll try to start over."

Choking back tears I said, "That's what I needed to hear, the encouragement I needed to start my next project." I was determined to help Joe stay in the dairy business by setting up a relief fund.

One of my partners in the veterinary practice, Dr. Ben, and I had already discussed how we wanted to help Joe if he committed to continue in the dairy business. We kick-started it by calling the North Carolina Department of Agriculture and getting their help in setting up a tax-exempt charitable entity called the "Joe Fund." Dr. Ben and I operated a dairy of our own in the Apex, North Carolina area, so we gave the first donation of a milking cow. We wrote all of our clients detailing the tragic events at Joe's farm and informed them of the "Joe Fund." The North Carolina Department of Agriculture spread the word to many other dairies in North Carolina.

The contributions started rolling in. Individual dairymen from North Carolina, South Carolina, and Virginia donated about 70 cows, delivering them directly to Joe's farm. Milk processing plants in North Carolina gave cash donations. Joe was able to borrow enough additional money to purchase 20 cows. Within a couple of weeks, he was back milking a similar-sized herd to what he owned before the poisoning. Joe thanked us profusely for our efforts and said he could not express how much this meant to him. However, Joe did find a way. A gift arrived by mail at Christmas time at both Dr. Ben's and my homes. Inside was a brass key chain with the inscription "24 Karat Friend."

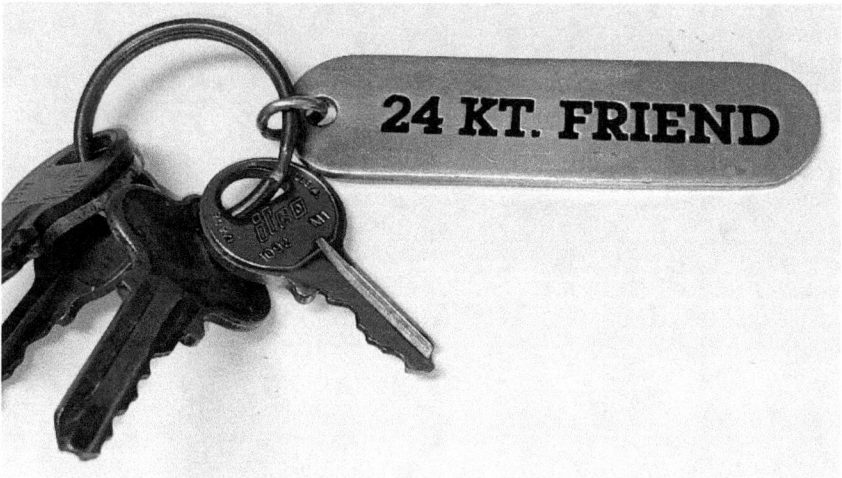

CHAPTER 15
Polarity Reversal in Kentucky

I received a telephone call late one evening that was quite unusual. A dairyman, Mr. Lake, and his brother in Kentucky were having serious problems with mastitis (udder infections) for over six months. The problem was about to put them out of business with the cost of treatment, loss of milk from antibiotic withholding, and excessive selling of affected cows. The dairyman called me not for help resolving the problem but to find out if the cows could have had a hidden mastitis problem when they purchased them six months ago. Could that problem have persisted for this long? Mr. Lake explained that he understood me to be the herd veterinarian at the farm that sold the cows, and he wanted to know if my client had sold him infected animals. The client who sold him the cows was my close friend Doug Child in Virginia.

You may recall from another story in this book that Doug had an exceptional all-registered herd of Holstein (black and white) cows. His herd was at the forefront of genetics in the breed, and it was a source of bulls for national breeding studs. Doug was an exceptional manager and did not have any unusual herd problems, or he could not have reached the elite level of being a genetic foundation herd. I called Doug the next morning to discuss the unusual phone call. Doug was surprised and saddened that the Lake brothers were having difficulties. He wanted to help them and even offered to pay any fees I incurred in resolving the problems. I assured him that it should not be necessary and that I would respond to them and investigate further if they needed help.

When I responded to Mr. Lake he was audibly very emotional. He could not make his payments to the bank for the loans the brothers had taken out to build a dairy barn and buy the cows when starting the business. They had only milked the cows for about a year and because of the mastitis they had lost a lot of money. They were about to lose everything—their land, buildings, equipment, and cows. There was already a date set for the cattle sale. He sounded very disheartened. I felt compelled to help in any way possible, so I began to take a detailed history over the phone.

The Lake brothers milked in an older facility for three months after they bought the new cows. During these three months, there were no cases of mastitis, but milking took too much time. After a new barn was completed, they moved into the new faster milk barn and began experiencing increasing mastitis cases. They called the equipment installer for help numerous times, but the company could find no problems with the equipment. Their veterinarian had cultured some of the affected cows and called the organism an environmental Streptococcus. The organism was easily treated with antibiotics but the milk had to be discarded during treatment and for several days after treatment.

Eventually, there were so many cows affected that milk discards almost equaled the milk sales. I asked if they had any printouts of milking equipment testing, and they said they were only given hand-written records of vacuum levels in the milking units and lines. There were no electronic graphs done while they watched, and they watched everything. They kept detailed records of all clinical cases, and they had monthly milk weights and records on each cow through DHIA (Dairy Herd Improvement Association).

I asked the Lake brothers to authorize my access to the computerized DHIA records and send me copies of all the laboratory testing and case records. Next I instructed them to call another milking equipment company and ask for a National Mastitis Council (NMC) equipment test and send me copies of the results. The requested data arrived at my office over the next two to three weeks. My analysis of the records and tests led me to a diagnosis that the equipment installed in the new barn was malfunctioning.

I had trained myself to evaluate milking equipment through the National Mastitis Council and various short courses taught by milking equipment manufacturers. It was a regular practice for me to do annual NMC evaluations on many of my dairy clients' milking systems as a mastitis preventive measure. I also operated a milking equipment supply company at the veterinary practice in order to renovate faulty systems, so I was very familiar with numerous types of milking equipment. I narrowed the problem at the Lake brothers' dairy down to the pulsator for the milking system and asked them to have the pulsators replaced.

When they did this, they were to send me an old pulsator for testing. They were also to report to me the following week about what their impression of the changing of pulsators had on the milking process and on the mastitis problem. The next week they telephoned and related that they were amazed at how much better the cows milked out and that they had not experienced any new mastitis cases. As a result of my findings and the response of the cows to the changes, I instructed them to engage a lawyer for help in recovering damages resulting from the equipment problem.

The Lake brothers followed all my instructions, and I was soon contacted by an attorney licensed in Kentucky. He gave me a quick interview and contracted with me for expert testimony services. So, the legal games began with the Lake brothers as plaintiffs and the milking equipment installer and the equipment manufacturer as defendants. The Lake brothers had to show three things: that there was a problem, that the Lakes sustained damages, and that the damages were caused by the accused defendants. The Lake brothers' lawyer was relying on me to help prove these points.

Justice is sometimes slow, and as a result, the bank forced the Lake brothers to sell their cows and equipment before the legal case was well underway. This was disturbing to me and devastating to the Lakes. I had hoped there was a way to keep this family in the food production business. Nevertheless, we proceeded to work on recovering damages. However, now the damages or economic losses included all the cows and the milking equipment, a sum close to a quarter of a million dollars.

The milking equipment manufacturer was a large international company and did not take being sued very well. They had many specialized lawyers, and they mounted a tough defense, hiring the best-known dairy experts in the United States. Their experts testified that the DHIA (Dairy Herd Improvement Association) records did not support the claim that there ever was a problem. When a cow has mastitis, there is infection and inflammation in the udder, increasing the white blood cells in the milk to fight the infection. DHIA milk testing detects the level of white blood cells in the milk and reports this monthly.

The Lakes' DHIA records never showed an elevated white cell count in the milk on test day. I countered their experts' claim by analyzing the individual cow records that are the source data of the computerized records. The Lake brothers were so diligent in identifying the affected cows that they always had them out of the milking string being treated, and therefore, discarded the milk when the DHIA supervisor came to test the herd. The milk of affected cows was never included in the DHIA-tested milk because of the presence of antibiotics. Consequently the elevated white cells were not represented in the test day data.

The detailed treatment records kept by the Lake brothers also verified what was done on DHIA test day with the treated cows held out of the test. Additionally, daily milk shipment totals were much lower than DHIA totals because the Lakes never shipped antibiotic-contaminated milk, even though DHIA estimated milk produced for all the cows. If one is confused by all of these statements, the bottom line is this: my analysis effectively countered their experts' assertions and established that there was a mastitis problem. Score one point for the Lake brothers.

Damages or economic losses were not hard to show, because we had a record of the lost milk, the treatment costs, and the fact that there was a forced sale of the cows and equipment. Of course, the cows were the recently purchased, high genetic value, registered cows from my friend Doug in Virginia. At the bank's forced sale, the milk cows did not bring anywhere near what their purchase price had been. The majority of the economic losses were from the forced sale. Since there was no way the defendants' lawyers could make the forced sale go away; they had to accept the damages calculated. Score point two for the Lake brothers.

We were left with the third and most crucial point to prove—that the damages were the result of the defendants' products or actions. Earlier, I analyzed the NMC (National Mastitis Council) milking system evaluation and testing protocol on the Lake brothers' milking system. I saw on the pulsator graphs that the installed pulsators were not opening fully and providing the necessary massage to the cows during milking. My suspicion was that the installer had not been properly trained by the manufacturer and had reversed the electrical polarity on the pulsators. In other words, he had put the wires on backward. The only way I could be sure was to test the pulsator myself and check to see if it had been magnetized by running backward.

Thankfully, I had the brothers send me an affected pulsator before the equipment was put in the forced sale. It checked out as I suspected, and was found to be magnetized. I would have to demonstrate this electrical problem to the jury to show how it could cause mastitis. The Lake brothers' lawyer was not sure how to do this. I told him I would need to milk a cow for the jury to show the incorrect milking of a magnetized pulsator. He could not envision taking a jury to a dairy farm nor bringing a cow into the courtroom. So, I suggested that I would build a portable milking machine using the magnetized pulsator, and I would also create an artificial udder that would demonstrate the milk flow problem that causes the mastitis.

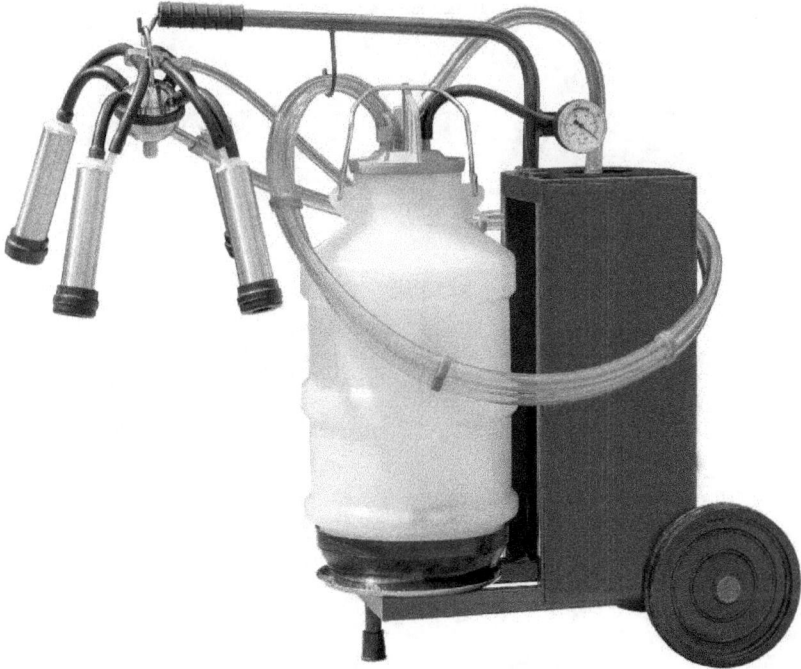

Example of a portable milking machine.

He was elated and shared this with the judge and the defendant's lawyers. The defendants' attorneys were livid. They didn't know that I possessed one of the damaged pulsators, and they had never been put in a position where they would have damaged equipment demonstrated to a jury. They objected to the plan, but the judge would have none of it. The judge said, "We could milk a cow on the courthouse lawn if need be."

Most legal cases are settled long before they get to trial. However, there was no movement on a settlement in this case up until the day of trial. I had packed my suitcase and loaded the portable milking machine and artificial udder into my pickup truck for the drive to Kentucky when a terrible winter storm hit and blanketed the state with ice. The Kentucky Highway Patrol closed all the roads. I telephoned the Lake brothers' lawyer for instructions on what to do about the travel restrictions, but could only leave a message. Later that day, he returned my call and told me that the defendants had agreed to settle the suit for the full amount of our demands rather than try to travel to Kentucky and milk a cow on the frozen courthouse lawn. My friend Doug and I had quite a chuckle over this!

CHAPTER 16
Lack of "A" Causes Many Problems

Mr. Fred Jaques and I had been friends since high school. We were from the same community in South Carolina and even played on high school sports teams together. We lost touch for several years while I went to vet school and spent time in the military. But, we reconnected when I started traveling to my family's farm in South Carolina after my father's death. Fred always wanted to farm, so to prepare for that career he decided to attend the state agricultural school and earned a degree in Agricultural Engineering. He was a successful swine and row crop farmer, but mostly desired a dairy farm. He eventually scraped together enough capital to buy used dairy equipment and installed it himself in buildings that he built himself. He bought young dairy heifers or baby dairy calves and raised them on land that had been in his family. It was a slow process, but the way he did it allowed him to get into the dairy business without the tremendous debt that most dairies carry. You can tell from these comments that I had a lot of admiration for Fred. It excited me when he called me to help with his veterinary work. For years when I traveled to South Carolina monthly to help my mother; I would schedule veterinary visits to his dairy herd and several others in the area.

After a few years of just routine reproduction checks, strange health problems began to appear in Fred's dairy herd. Even though his herd was mostly young, the cows began to move slowly, as if their feet hurt or they were weak. Some of the cows would develop pustular abscesses deep in the muscles that would not heal. An abnormally high number of cows developed eye lesions. I primarily did reproductive work for Fred's herd, and it became hard to get cows pregnant. It took too many breedings to get a conception, and this was not the usual situation for Fred, who did all of the artificial breeding.

He reluctantly purchased a "clean up" bull to improve the breeding rate. Milk production began to decrease, and profits were pinched. Several of these same problems began to occur on some of the other herds I served in the area. It became perplexing to the dairymen, and they shared their observations with each other. I recognized the frustration in my friend Fred and convinced him to let me investigate using labs and other means at my disposal. He not only agreed to let me look further at his farm, but contacted the other dairymen in the area he had been talking with. Five farms all opened their herds and records to the investigation.

Record reviews revealed that most of the dairies were experiencing similar unusual health problems; some more, some less than Fred. An epidemiological survey was begun. There was very little common between the various dairies. They all grew their own forages for feeding the cows on their own land. None of the farms were really close to each other. They had separate wells. All the farms had closed herds meaning they didn't buy and sell cattle and they all raised their own herd replacement heifers on their separate farms. They all had their own labor and didn't share employees. They all had good vaccination and disease prevention programs but used widely different commercially prepared health products. They all had different rations and combinations of feeds, with one exception. There was an obvious commonality: all the dairy farms bought a grain mix from the same feed company.

Another veterinarian from the local area, Dr. Riley, was also trying to understand the problems he was seeing in his client's herds. We joined our resources and began to analyze various blood samples and feeds from the herds. The blood parameters were compared to known normal cow blood levels for a variety of vitamins and minerals. The analyzed feed nutrient levels were compared to the levels specified on each farm's computer ration specifications generated by the feed company. The other veterinarian handled most of the blood analysis, and I performed the diagnostic ration analyses because of my nutrition training. Almost simultaneously, we both detected low vitamin A levels in blood samples and feed samples.

Low blood vitamin A was totally unexpected because all of these farms were paying to have higher stress levels of vitamins added to their feeds, due to the heat stress of the southeastern summer. Vitamin A deficiency symptoms include reduced reproductive efficiency, abortions, eye lesions, impaired immunity with increased rates of infections, poor bone growth, and reduced feed intake. Many of these symptoms were observed on each of the cooperating dairies, so the clinical signs at the farms fit the laboratory findings of low vitamin A. We were pretty sure that our epidemiologic survey had found the etiology (cause) of the herd problems. However, at this juncture, we had no clue as to why the feed levels of vitamin A did not meet the specifications prescribed by the ration printouts.

I gathered all of the computer ration printouts of the cooperating dairies and listed the feed company's guaranteed levels of Vitamin A in the grain and mineral mixes. Then I compared them to the laboratory analysis levels. Any farm-purchased feed analysis data that was missing from the list was resampled and analyzed at the same laboratory as the original samples. The results were amazingly consistent in that none of the samples met the Vitamin A levels guaranteed by the feed company. I telephoned the feed company, but no one at the feed mill would answer my questions. The company responded through its lawyers, so it was time for my dairy friends to lawyer up. They all chose to be represented by the same law firm, partly because it was a small community and partly because the firm never lost cases in that county.

Our firm's senior partner had been a state senator and had helped everyone in the community at some time. That meant anyone who could serve on a jury owed the firm a favor. As a result, I felt confident that the feed company would cooperate with us to further investigate this problem. Our attorneys assigned me the task of accessing the damages, so I requested two weeks to pour over all the cow and production records from the five farms.

The damages were substantial because almost three thousand cows were owned by the five farms, and the health-related problems had occurred for many months. After the damages were calculated, our lawyers hired me to further investigate the feed mill and try to determine how the low vitamin levels had occurred. The feed company continued to cooperate with us.

Feed mills purchase vitamins in concentrate form and they are added in precisely weighed quantities to tons of other ingredients to make a finished feed. I spent most of a day watching the mixing and weighing procedures, checking scale accuracies, and pulling samples. Then I sent these pulled samples to the same feed laboratory we had been using. Puzzlingly, nothing manufactured that day fell outside of expected feed specification levels. This meant that the mill was capable of correctly manufacturing feeds.

With the revelation that the feed mill could accurately manufacture feeds, our attorneys suspected that there was perhaps a purposeful omission of nutrients from the feeds. A lawsuit was then filed so that the lawyers could question the feed company personnel under oath. These questioning sessions are called depositions and are taken under oath for admission later as evidence in the courtroom proceedings. On the day of the depositions, the feed company's head nutritionist admitted that he purposely reduced the Vitamin A levels. He did this because it saved the company money, and in his opinion, he didn't think the higher levels were necessary. I don't think he actually did this solely out of company loyalty, but he took the fall for it. I guess this demonstrates the accuracy of the old saying, "The truth is at the end of the money trail."

For our attorneys, these actions resulted in fraudulent guarantees on the computer feed printouts. Thankfully, the feed company liability insurer, who was present at the depositions, had heard enough and was willing to settle the case without any further proof that vitamin levels actually caused all the problems. The out-of-court settlement paid that very day was for millions of dollars allocated to each of the dairies, according to my damages estimates. All of these farms were able to use their settlements to fully recover and stay in the business of producing food—a win for the dairy farms and a win for my passion for feeding people. Fred, my childhood friend, was so pleased with the outcome that we continued a lifelong friendship and professional relationship. We saw each other almost every month for 30 years until we both retired.

CHAPTER 17
Saving 300 Million in Italy

The Open Grounds Farm first described in the story about a "quick burst of speed" was owned by a giant Italian agricultural company. Actually, it was owned by an Italian family called the Feruzzi Group. I thought when I began working at Open Grounds that it was the grandest farm I had ever seen. But, as the years went by and I got close to some important people in the farm's management, they revealed the enormity of the whole agricultural enterprise.

The Feruzzi Group had holdings and properties all over the world. The company owned and managed over two million acres of farms and many agriculture-related commodity businesses. The Feruzzi Group was the second largest company in Italy behind the Fiat Auto Group, owned by the Agnelli family.

I picked up a great opportunity when Livio, the manager at Open Grounds Farm, was promoted to worldwide farm manager for the Feruzzi Group. He and I had worked closely together for several years and we had gained a lot of trust in and respect for each other. We had actually become close friends through our Open Grounds Farm relationship.

Livio was exceptionally talented. He was fluent in at least four languages to the extent that he could read and understand scientific literature in those languages. He had a doctorate in agronomy and understood crop and beef cattle farming both technically and economically. However, he lacked experience in the modern dairy industry. He knew I had specialized in dairy herd production medicine and even owned and operated two dairies in North Carolina myself. So, he asked me to help him with dairy supervision decisions within the Feruzzi Group. I was thrilled with the prospect of expanding my work with this company.

My first opportunity to help Livio with a dairy decision came within a year of his promotion. The Feruzzi Group owned a large farm in northeast Italy near Trieste called Torvis. Torvis grew many commodities such as soybeans, sugar beets, and corn but it also had three operating dairies and a milk processing plant. One dairy was 800 cows, another was 200 cows, and the third dairy was 600 cows in milk. Livio asked me to travel to Italy and evaluate the dairies, with the ultimate purpose of the trip being to make recommendations on expanding one of the dairy's cattle housing areas. The cost of the expansion was about 300 million lire. This sounded like a lot of money to me.

Well, I never thought I would ever leave the United States so I didn't quite know where to start. My wife, however, loved traveling and she had great ideas about where to start. I could start by taking her with me to Italy. Seriously though, she was a big help and it just so happened that we were celebrating a big tenth wedding anniversary that year, so it was a no-brainer to take her. We excitedly applied for passports and began to gather things together for our first trip abroad. My mother was happy to stay with our children while we were traveling.

Livio asked me what the work would cost the company and I confessed that I had no idea what to charge, because I didn't know anything about what the trip would cost me. I suggested that I would do this for free if the Feruzzi Group would let me take my wife, pay all our expenses, and give us a few days of travel around Italy to see their beautiful country. Livio quickly agreed to the terms. I really knew little about this company and I had no concept of the fantastic treatment which we would receive from them during the trip.

The day of departure came soon. I had never left North America so I was very excited. Our flight would go from Raleigh to Munich, Germany and then we would take a commuter flight over the Alps to Trieste, Italy. The flight to Munich was uneventful, however, at Munich things got a little more exciting. When we changed to the commuter flight terminal we saw armored vehicles and many armed soldiers guarding the airport and its gates. Germany had been the recent target of terrorists and the German government was not having any more of it. Security was tight. I had purchased a new computer for the trip called a Panasonic Sr. Partner. It was state of the art at the time, weighing a mere 38 pounds and sporting a built-in thermal printer, a green screen, and an expansive eight-inch floppy disk drive.

The German security had never seen anything like this totally modern portable computer, so it immediately created suspicion. I tried to explain to the guards what all the features were, but they weren't sure of what I said due to the language barrier. They insisted I turn it on, however, my power converter was in the checked luggage, and I had hand-carried my valuable computer. I knew Europe was on a different power grid but I never anticipated that I should hand-carry the power converter. The guards did not have a converter and they said it was impossible to find my luggage with my converter. I insisted that I could not leave the computer. So, a guard with an automatic weapon took me aside and into a room with the computer. My wife had to wait outside.

Inside the room another guard handed me a screwdriver and told me to take it apart. For fear of being arrested, I began to take the brand-new computer apart. I managed to remove all the covers, and when the guards saw that there was no bomb inside the strange box, they allowed me to replace the covers and rejoin my wife. At last, we were allowed to board our final flight. We almost missed it!

I was glad to arrive in Trieste, Italy, and see my name on a chauffeur's sign. We followed the gentleman to his car and were driven to a fine old hotel in the historic part of the city. The evening meal was quite an event. When I attempted to decipher the Italian lire prices, which ran into the tens of thousands, we were advised by our waiter, who astonishingly was waiting solely on us, that the Feruzzi family already paid for everything. Of course, I could not read the Italian menu, so I asked our waiter to order for us. The food kept coming and coming. It was delicious, and I hurt myself that night. The next morning we found espresso and cakes delivered to our room. At about nine o'clock, we ventured down to the lobby to meet the Torvis farm host and begin the work portion of the trip.

Surprisingly, the farm host was accompanied by a cute, young, bilingual, Italian girl who was to be my wife's tour guide for the day. They quickly connected and left for the sights in Trieste. I rode along with my farm host, who was a bilingual, young, Italian man with training in agronomy. He would be my translator for the farm visit. When we arrived at the farm, he took me straight into the office of the farm manager, Mr. Prosperi. Mr. Prosperi was a well-dressed, important-looking man who was a protégé of my friend Dr. Livio.

After exchanging niceties through the translator, he asked me what I would like to see. I told him I wished to see everything dairy related. I needed to understand everything in order to advise properly about the building of a new barn that could cost over 300 million lire.

I dove right into the job by gathering data, translating the metric measures into American measures, and writing all of this in my little notebook. I measured every area and made notes on everything from bedding types to feeding and milking techniques for all three separate dairies at Torvis. The first dairy I toured and evaluated was a large 800 cow dairy with housing in straw-bedded individual free stalls. Individual freestalls are setup to hold one cow comfortably and the cows are free to choose any stall that appeals to them. This group of cows was milked on a carrousel or round, rotating platform. As the carrousel turned, an opening appeared for a cow to enter. She stepped onto the platform and was individually prepared for milking by one operator. By the time she rode all the way around the barn, she was milked and allowed to step off to return to her housing area. I was amazed that the cows knew how to do all of this.

The second dairy was a small 200-cow dairy with housing in a straw-bedded lounging pack barn. These cows were not confined to one free stall but were allowed to mingle in a large bedded pack area. They were milked in an old, slow milk barn with eight individual manually operated gated stalls. The cows were prepared for milking one at a time by an individual operator. After completing milking, they returned to their loose housing area. I was really enjoying learning about these dairies and the history of the farm and region. It surprised me that the farm was developed by Benito Mussolini, who, as it turns out, was quite an agriculturalist before he was hanged for getting Italy into World War Two on the wrong side.

By the time we finished touring the first two dairies, it was noon, and the group wanted to take me to a favorite trattoria (restaurant). So, I tucked my tape measure and my little notebook away for a while. The meal was very delicious, and after last night I had learned to pace myself. But I can't say the same for my hosts, especially about the wine. Everyone was really having a good time, so much so that my young translator told me he was drunk and I'd be on my own for the afternoon. Poor guy, he was so embarrassed.

Nonetheless, I finally convinced the group that we should leave, so that I could see the last and most important dairy in the daylight. It was this last dairy that was asking for the new housing barn. The 600 cows in the last dairy rested in a large loose housing area on a straw-bedded pack, much like the smallest dairy, only the housing was much larger for the larger groups. The cows were milked in a new state-of-the-art double 24 herringbone design milking parlor. The cows came into the barn in groups of 24 at a time and stood side by side. This meant that the cows were handled for milking preparation in groups of 24 instead of individually as in the two other milking barns.

Only when the last cow in the group was prepped and milked could the group leave, so there was a mad rush to get the cows prepped. The prepping of the cows in the two other barns was done one at a time without rushing the chore. In this barn, the prep was so rushed it was dangerously lacking in sanitation. After measuring the housing spaces and noting the differences in milking technique, I was ready to look at the new building plans.

A draftsman drew the plans and it was easy for me to convert them to American measurements. I quickly made the conversions. Then it was time for me to ask some questions.

"What are you trying to accomplish with the new barn?" I asked. "You will not be increasing the milking herd size," I stated.

The farm personnel then answered, "The herd veterinarian recommended the new barn to give the cows more room and decrease the mastitis in the herd."

I had suspected there was a mastitis problem here in this barn because I had recorded the milk quality data for each dairy in my little notebook. I also recorded my observations of the rushed milking preparation. I was surprised that the Torvis management would plan a 300 million lire building project based solely on the conjecture by a veterinarian that it would reduce mastitis. This is why the clever Livio sent me to Torvis! He did not send me to evaluate the building plans. He sent me to evaluate the reason for the building.

I did my best to explain to the farm personnel that the building would not solve the mastitis problem, but I needed to have my translator with me and he was not able to attend after the lively lunch. I decided to wait until the next day and take the plans back to the hotel for an in-depth review before I shared my planned strategy with Mr. Prosperi through my translator.

The next morning with my translator present, I showed Mr.

Prosperi that all the housing areas had the same square meters per cow for lounging. The new proposed barn also had the identical same space per cow, not more. Therefore, there would be no increase in space. I pointed out that the smallest dairy had the lowest mastitis rate and it had the same type of housing as the 600 cow dairy with the highest mastitis problem. Then I described the differences in milking preparation at the three dairies and the impact that the poor preparation was having at the 600 cow dairy.

He had a skeptical look on his face, so I took him with me to all the dairies to demonstrate the points I had made. Finally, I gave Mr. Prosperi a preferred milking technique for the 600 cow dairy and challenged him to use this technique for three months before considering a new building. All of this information was put in a report to Livio when I returned to the United States. To my knowledge, 35 years later, the barn never had to be built. But, now for the rest of the story of my first trip to Italy.

After our time in Trieste the Feruzzi Group moved us to Venice for two days. We stayed in a four-star hotel on the Grand Canal just down from the Feruzzi house located on the Grand Canal. We had a splendidly romantic gondola ride with a singing Italian pilot. We walked all over the city admiring the architecture and visiting numerous museums as well as other tourist spots. We dined in excellent four-star restaurants, and we were not allowed to even leave a tip. Next, we were transported to Rome and met a friend of my wife who lived and worked in Rome. He gave us the tour of a lifetime. We had so much fun with him that we made it a point to connect with him several more times on future visits to Rome.

I had studied Latin in school and read much about Rome and its history. To be able to see the things I read about in person made a lasting impression on me, and Rome became my favorite city in the world. Italian food became my favorite food, and Italian people became some of my favorite people. In subsequent years I made many more trips to Italy, at least one per year, and many of those trips were with Livio. I owe the Feruzzi family a great debt of gratitude for broadening my worldview and inspiring me to support food production around the globe. Perhaps I made a down payment on this debt when I saved them 300 million.

CHAPTER 18
Coughing and Breaking Bones in Carolina

Mr. Daniels was a longtime client of our North Carolina veterinary practice. He appeared to be very successful in his dairy business and was always expanding his cow numbers. He had moved his whole herd from a small farm to a larger farm several years before I joined the practice and he had been increasing his herd size every year. It was not long after I moved to North Carolina that I became the practice partner primarily responsible for this client. Mr. Daniels was important to us because he used many of the services we offered to our clients. He used us for reproductive exams monthly, his farm used some of the milking equipment we offered, he used us for sick animal care, he bought many veterinary supplies, and he used our nutritional consulting services.

His dairy was local to us, and we really did our best to provide him with good client service. However, Mr. Daniels was like numerous dairymen with years of experience; he treated many of his animals himself out of convenience and economy. So, it surprised me following a herd pregnancy exam visit when he detained me and asked if I could look at some calves he had been treating for pneumonia after hearing some coughing in the group. I, of course, jumped at the opportunity to help.

We drove to a nearby farm where he housed, fed, and managed his young stock. I was shown a group of about 120 young growing calves four to six months old. He had sent his help on ahead to catch a few of the sick calves so that my time would be used efficiently. There was a little coughing in the group, but none of them looked particularly sick. He put a few of them into a lane leading to a head catch so that I could safely examine them. My thermometer revealed a mild fever in a few of the calves so I began to question Mr. Daniels about his treatment process and therapeutic products. He was using a commonly available over-the-counter antibiotic given daily intramuscularly by injection.

I suggested changing to a longer-acting antibiotic given under the skin. I recommended this for two reasons. One was for labor efficiency, only treating every three days. Secondly, I noticed several calves limping, causing me to suspect muscle damage from frequent or improper injections. I noticed the calves limping only on the back legs, usually the right rear. Mr. Daniels corrected my assumption by telling me that they had not treated any of these calves yet, and there were dozens of them limping for some unknown reason. He explained further that most of the limping calves were lying down in a nearby open-sided barn.

I walked over to the barn to examine some of the calves and found that all of them had broken legs. I asked if there had been a larger animal in the group that may have injured these calves, but he had no explanation for the injuries. I began to suspect a feeding problem, but how could this happen? I did their nutritional work. I was as capable of making a mistake as any consultant, so I pulled feed samples and recorded the numbers of the affected calves. I told them to only treat calves that were coughing or showed nasal discharges and had a fever, so as to limit the numbers being handled until we found the reason for the lameness.

I hurried back to my office to re-analyze my last nutritional recommendations. I spent hours looking over the rations and found nothing wrong. Calcium and phosphorus are the main minerals in bone development, and the dietary levels and ratios of calcium to phosphorus are important for gut absorption of these minerals. No recommendations fell outside of the specifications of one point five to two point five to one (1.5-2.5:1) calcium to phosphorus. In other words, I could find nothing wrong in my work.

I thought maybe we were dealing with something else until the next day when Mr. Daniels called and told me a calf had become paralyzed while catching it in the head gate. They were taking the calf to the North Carolina Diagnostic Laboratory. The laboratory called later that day and told me the calf had crushed a neck vertebra and damaged the spinal cord. It was such a strange injury that the lab veterinarian looked further and found the skull to be thin and found leg bones and other vertebrae to be thin, as if to be demineralized. I knew then that there was some ration problem, but how could it be?

A new ration formulation was made that increased the calcium to the highest level and widest ratio safe for feeding in order to compensate for the bone demineralization. I scheduled an appointment with Mr. Daniels to review this change and traveled to his farm. He thanked me for the recommendations and informed me that he had found the problem. I had made feed mix formulas for him in 1,000 batch sizes because 1,000 pound formulas were easily scalable to larger batches. His mix-mill could make a 10,000 pound batch, so he scaled up all the ingredients, except he overlooked the calcium source. Since he didn't scale up the calcium source, it was being fed at one-tenth the recommended amount. I was very relieved that I had not caused his troubles, and I emphasized that he should feed the new formula for several weeks until we were sure the bones had all re-mineralized.

As I drove away from the farm, I felt some weight off of my shoulders, but this feeling was short-lived. Snow and sleet were falling and covering the ground with an icy sheet. The paved roads were warm, so they were not accumulating ice. But the pastures were becoming skating rinks. The whole next week I worried about the calves and the possibility of more broken bones on the slick pastures. Fortunately, the men at Mr. Daniels' farm were expert cattlemen, and there were no more broken bones or new cases of pneumonia. Over the next months, the ration changes healed the calves, and they entered the milking herd on schedule. A sizable economic loss was averted mostly because a few calves in a group started coughing and drew our attention.

CHAPTER 19
Acid Indigestion in a Thousand

Cows are ruminants and have a very unique digestive system as was mentioned in the introductory chapters. Ruminants have their stomach divided into four compartments. There are three (before) forestomachs and one true stomach similar to the stomach in monogastrics like people. The forestomachs are really large fermentation vats where friendly microbes digest and utilize the ruminant's high fiber forage diet. The ruminant provides the microbes with a warm, moist environment that is frequently refilled with new food, mixed, and kept at a safe, constant pH or acidity.

There is a delicate balance between the ruminant animal and its microbes that can be dangerously upset, particularly when the acidity is not controlled. When cattle are given access to too much grain or starch, there is rapid fermentation of the starch to lactic acid, which upsets the acid balance in the forestomachs. Some of the rumen microbes can then overgrow and produce large amounts of acid which kills other microbe populations and leads to stomach wall damage, liver abscesses, and a condition called laminitis.

Laminitis occurs when the acid in the stomach produces inflammatory products that make blood pool in the feet and diminish the oxygen supply to the important lamina tissue that binds foot tissues together. Laminitis is very painful for cows and is life-threatening because they will not get up to eat or drink. My ruminant nutrition degree program was all about properly balancing the grain and forage percentages in the diet to avoid a life-threatening acid shift in the rumen. Not all people feeding cows are adequately aware of the problems they can cause when they try to push production higher by feeding too much grain. I give you this information because it is the

95

basic physiology involved in several herd problems that I had to identify and manage.

Regrettably, this case report is about Mr. Daniels's dairy farm from the preceding story. A little additional background is necessary to frame the situation. I had done the nutrition work at the Daniels farm for years until I made the decision to leave the large group practice at Apex, North Carolina, and start a solo (by myself) practice. When I made this change, I was bound by a non-compete agreement with the practice that prevented my working with former clients for a few years. The decision to leave the former clients and friends was very difficult; however, for me to expand my efforts towards global food supply services, it was a necessary intermediate step. I would be able to return to many of these former clients if they so desired at a future date.

In this particular problem investigation, I was not called in by Mr. Daniels. I was advising a multinational company marketing a novel milk production enhancement product to the dairy industry, and that company requested for me to investigate problems at the Daniels farm. The company had received information that the Daniels herd was having too many health problems to safely use their new product. The Daniels farm had expanded to milk over one –thousand cows daily. It was among the largest and most visible farms in the Carolinas, so Mr. Daniels was perceived to be a potentially important and visible customer.

Additionally, before I could get a visit scheduled, I was contacted by another multinational company that marketed frozen cattle semen for artificial insemination. This company related that their technicians were having difficulty getting cows pregnant at the Daniels farm and that this low success was highly unusual considering the high success of the past years. This second multinational company wanted me to investigate the breeding at the Daniels farm. Therefore, my investigation was funded by multinational companies. As a result the Daniels had no cost in the investigative work done.

When I arrived, I was totally surprised by the change in the state of affairs at the farm from the time when I had known them a few years before. The observation and information-gathering process for this large dairy took most of a day, and I'll make a quick listing of the steps involved. The investigation began with us renewing our previous friendship and reviewing the history for each of us during the years of absence.

I was then given a tour of their new larger facilities. I walked through the numerous pens of cattle, noting excessive body condition, sporadic diarrhea, and many lame cows. I was given the opportunity to review the herd DHIA records which revealed low milk production levels and low milk butterfat percentages. I next made copies of feeding recommendations. Lastly, I was taken to a group of 150 cows that were outside on a pasture, unable to walk to the dairy barn to be milked any more than once daily because their feet hurt too badly. This outside hospital group represented almost fifteen percent of the milking herd.

At the Daniels' request, I telephoned their local veterinarian, and he begged for relief from multiple trips per week for emergency digestive upset treatments. After only one day on the farm, I was suspicious that the herd was experiencing acidosis from feeding too much grain, but I would need time to analyze the feeding programs to be certain.

That evening in my home office, I used my computer to "back" into the ration and did an analysis of the feeds and feeding rates prescribed for the cows. The feed company did not give the farm the ration printouts with nutrient specifications, so I was required to do a ration calculation in reverse. In nutritional evaluations, we always run our calculations on a dry matter basis which is a method of looking at the nutrients and nutrient requirements equalized at zero moisture content. I converted all the feedstuffs to dry matter equivalents and performed the diagnostic ration analysis.

The ration was dangerously high in grains and grain byproducts; 70 percent of the ration dry matter was from expensive grain-type feeds supplied by the feed company. The remainder of the ration was from less expensive farm-raised corn silage or forage. As a result, the daily feed cost was excessively high. In the herds that I feed, I try to have a grain-to-forage ratio of around 40 to 45 percent grain and 55 to 60 percent forage. The Daniels were being told to feed a 70 percent grain to 30 percent forage ratio feed mix.

This was the reason for so many digestive upsets, bloats, lameness, poor milking performance, and poor reproductive performance. I returned to the Daniels farm the next day to explain my findings and discovered, to my amazement, that they were already aware of the problems and the causes. Oddly, they were just very afraid to say anything to the feed company representative about the dangerous feeding recommendations. Their fear had them paralyzed.

I was totally taken aback by the Daniels's feelings of helplessness from a feeding and a financial standpoint. It was explained that the state government had pushed them to build new facilities to meet newly created waste management regulations. This construction project was so expensive that it required them to expand the milk cow numbers to pay for the new facilities. They were left with a large debt that they would need to finance.

Additionally, during the construction process, the traditional farm industry banks slow-walked their funding requests, thereby creating a funding shortfall that forced the Daniels to seek emergency funds from alternative sources. The source of emergency funds that had the best financing was from the large feed company they were presently using. The deal that the feed company offered was to lend the Daniels funds as long as they would use only the feed company's feeds and consultants. This arrangement seemed innocuous at first, but soon the Daniels were feeding huge amounts of feed company grains and spending huge amounts for the grains.

The Daniels were afraid to challenge the situation for fear of losing their financing. I informed the Daniels that the contract offered by the feed company was illegal. It is referred to as a "tying arrangement" and was judged unenforceable years ago when fertilizer companies tried to take advantage of small farmers. I had prepared a safer, lower-cost ration for the herd using more of their farm-raised forages, and I encouraged them to feed it to a group of cows and monitor their production and health. The ration could save them a substantial amount, about $1.50 per cow per day compared to the present ration.

Two weeks later, I returned to the Daniels's dairy. Mr. Daniels had put the entire herd on my new ration. The milk production had come up a little already, and cows' feet were healing to the point that reproductive performance was improving. The best thing about the new ration was Mr. Daniels was saving $1.50 per cow per day on 1,000 cows. This amounted to $1,500 per day, or $45,000 per month, or over half a million dollars per year. With these numbers in his mind, Mr. Daniels was ready to take the gamble and challenge the feed company. He contacted a local attorney. I agreed to continue helping Mr. Daniels while his attorney handled the legal mess. In the meantime, I communicated with the companies that had paid for the herd investigation, and they were satisfied that the problems would eventually be resolved so that they could soon resume business with the farm as usual.

The herd continued to improve, and the attorneys continued to run up bills. From here, the story of the Daniels dairy takes a turn for the worse. Eventually, the feed company filed for bankruptcy and the local attorney, fearing he might never get paid, made a crooked deal with the feed company's attorneys to settle the case using cash for the lawyer and stock in the failing company for the Daniels dairy. In the settlement, the Daniels had to sell their cows, but they were able to keep the farm after filing for reorganization bankruptcy themselves. The only ones that came out of this situation whole were the lawyers. Because of the bankruptcy, at that time I was not even paid for the help I had given them during the legal proceedings.

Surprisingly however, I received a pleasant surprise months later in the form of a check for payment in full for my services. The Daniels were honest, hard-working people, and they, unknown to me, had filed a protective lien on my behalf. They truly appreciated the help I had given them. When the farm emerged from bankruptcy, the courts honored the protective lien and paid me in full. I still regret today that these fine people were put in a situation where government pressure, lender failure, feed company trickery, and lawyer crookedness denied them of their ability to make a profit in their chosen occupation of dairy production.

CHAPTER 20
Disappointing Startup in Carolina

Over the years I have worked alongside other veterinarians. I feel it is important to not always be "in competition" with other professionals, because it puts the farmers in the difficult position of feeling disloyal to their "regular vet" in order to get another opinion on their situation. Additionally, it is important to share knowledge and experience with younger professionals and students to encourage sustainable excellence in food production medicine. This attitude led to the referral of a case from a veterinarian friend and former partner, Dr. Ben Shelton, now practicing in western North Carolina.

Dr. Ben had a good client and close friend, Jeff, who operated a large one-thousand cow dairy and was suffering through very depressing herd problem. Dr. Ben feared his friend was almost at the point of doing something drastic because of a severe mastitis (udder infection) problem at the dairy. The problem had been very costly and Dr. Ben felt that there would need to be legal actions taken to recover the damages. Dr. Ben preferred not to get involved with the legal system, so he telephoned me on behalf of Jeff. Little did I know when I agreed to take on this challenge that it would result in the longest and most unusual legal mess that I would ever encounter.

I finally reached Mr. Jeff late one evening after trying to contact him at various times for two or three days. Jeff was a busy, hardworking dairyman who kept exceptionally long hours. We discussed his situation for several minutes on the phone until it became apparent that I needed to see and test the facility and look at his records to make much sense of the problem. A visit to his farm was set up for the following week.

What a state-of-the art facility this was! Mr. Jeff proudly gave me a walking tour of the farm. He showed me the cattle and their housing area where the cows were bedded in individual freestalls on sand bedding, the cleanest and most desirable bedding type. Fans for air movement were everywhere keeping cows cool and the environment dry. The cow lots were cleaned three times per day by a water flush system which was released while cows were in the milk barn. This was an ideal sanitation situation.

We next went into the milking barn, where an automatic gate gently kept the cows moving into the milking stalls. The stalls were arranged side by side in a herringbone pattern, eighteen on each side of a sunken pit where the milkmen worked. The milking parlor was very clean and quiet because the noisy equipment was in a basement beneath the barn. The milkmen quickly cleaned, sanitized, and dried the cows, preparing them for the milking units which were held by an arm of an automatic milker removal system. Cow udders were once again sanitized before they were let out to return to the freshly cleaned housing area.

Next, we went upstairs to the main office where computers were located. The computers identified each cow being milked and measured milk quantity and milk flow. The computers controlled the automatic milk unit removal system and tallied the daily production of each cow for reports. The computer would recognize when a cow's production deviated from normal and would flag her for managers to examine. "The technology in the system is amazing and expensive!" asserted Mr. Jeff.

Lastly, we went downstairs to the basement, where most of the mechanical components of the milking system were located. It was in this area that we spent the remainder of our time because this is where installation mistakes and equipment malfunctions were found that induced the severe herd mastitis problem. Mr. Jeff's expressions of pride changed to expressions of frustration as he showed me changes that he had made to reduce the mastitis incidence in the herd.

First he had to replace an expensive computer controlled vacuum pump costing $60,000 when it ejected water and sand in its exhaust. He had begun to experience increased mastitis levels at this time and changing the vacuum pump did not correct the spike in mastitis. The milking equipment manufacturer and the local installer came out together to the farm to perform equipment testing and said everything checked out well. As mastitis levels continued to rise and more cows started getting seriously ill, Mr. Jeff called his local vet Dr. Ben, and

Dr. Ben called in an independent milking system specialist.

This Texas-based specialist checked the system and found that it had never been properly evaluated by the well-respected National Mastitis Council testing protocol. (The National Mastitis Council was discussed in the previous story of "*No Holes Bored*".) The Texas specialist knew the evaluation had not been performed because he had to install all the needed test ports before he could do his evaluation. Mr. Jeff knew at this point that the local installer had never properly tested the new system.

The milking system specialist found that a large vacuum supply pipe had been improperly buried underground and had collapsed during construction, allowing vacuum leakage and vacuum instability which led to mastitis cases. The collapsed line also allowed sand and water to enter the vacuum line and damage the vacuum pump. In addition, in order to increase his profits the local installer substituted cheaper, inferior end-of-milking shut-off valves that were not the ones specified on the system blueprints. Initially, the equipment manufacturer did not know this substitution had been made but didn't change them when they found the substitution. These malfunctioning valves, along with the vacuum instability, caused severe mastitis and eventually cost Mr. Jeff many cows.

I documented everything as usual. I took videos and many notes and tested all the equipment. Then I retested the equipment with the old malfunctioning components back in the system to document the vacuum instability and restriction of milk flow which would contribute to mastitis. Lastly, I looked at all the records of milk bacterial testing and treatment that were in Dr. Ben's and Mr. Jeff's files. After a week of reviewing the herd visit findings and researching the connections concerning milking machine malfunctions as a cause of mastitis, I was ready to recommend to Mr. Jeff that he had good grounds for legal action against the milking equipment manufacturer and the installer. I asked Mr. Jeff to contact some local attorneys to handle the lawsuit and we could interview them on my next visit to his farm.

In the meantime, we made necessary changes to the milking system to correct the installation and equipment deficiencies. After vacuum supply lines were rerouted, the inferior shut-off valves were replaced, and a new vacuum pump was installed, the system was thoroughly evaluated for proper function by the National Mastitis Council protocols. Following the system corrections, the incidence of new mastitis cases rapidly decreased. This quick reversal of mastitis infections gave validity to our causation theories and corrective recommendations. Mr. Jeff's anxiety over the health of his cows was alleviated, and he began to once again enjoy his chosen work. Recovering some of his damages was the last bit of medicine needed to heal his business.

Mr. Jeff found only one law firm that was willing to take the case. As I look back now, they probably took the case because they didn't know anything about cattle mastitis or farm litigation. Since he didn't have any other choices, Mr. Jeff hired this small local firm to begin the suit. Over the next few weeks, papers were filed with the court, and the case moved along. Then everything on our lawyer's side stopped abruptly. Both the senior attorney and his junior partner were in the North Carolina National Guard, and they were both called to active duty in the Gulf War. They were shipped off to Iraq. They were there for almost a year, and the senior attorney even got injured while there. The law firm tried to keep up with things in their absence but struggled without enough experienced guidance.

In contrast to Mr. Jeff, the equipment manufacturer, had very deep pockets and hired high-priced, highly experienced lawyers that watched every detail. As would be the situation, a filing deadline was missed by our attorneys, and the opposing attorneys filed for and were granted a dismissal by the court. It appeared that all was lost as far as recovering damages from the installer and the equipment manufacturer. We could no longer sue them for their negligence and they got off Scott-free. Our attorneys had lost that opportunity for Mr. Jeff.

However, we did have the ability to file a suit against our attorneys for malpractice for missing a known, required filing date. The problem with this plan was we could not find an attorney willing to sue another attorney for malpractice even though attorneys have insurance for this purpose. It appears most attorneys use the same malpractice insurer and the insurance company frowns on being sued by someone they insure.

Before giving up on Mr. Jeff's damages recovery, I confided in an attorney friend of mine, Mr. Bryson, whom I knew through Boy Scouts of America. Mr. Bryson was a real justice warrior and recognized the unfairness of Mr. Jeff's situation. He agreed to take the case and help us. To his surprise, after doing some research on North Carolina law, he found that in order to prove legal malpractice, he would have to prove that the underlying case was winnable. This meant that he would have to litigate the original mastitis case and win it before the insurance company would pay any damages. What a convoluted mess!

The Lawyer's Mutual Insurance Company was responsible for defending our old law firm in the malpractice suit, so it hired the same high-powered, expensive lawyers that had represented the equipment manufacturer in the original mastitis damages case. This gave the opposition team all of the information from both sides of the previous case, an advantage that the insurance company was sure would tilt the scales of justice in their favor. Depositions (sworn testimony) of mastitis experts and fact witnesses began all over again. After another year or so of legal preparation and maneuvering, the case was finally on the court's schedule. Mr. Bryson had studied, questioned, and absorbed a tremendous amount of new knowledge about the disease mastitis and its relationship to management, environment, and milking machines. His legal team was ready for trial.

Fortunately for us, I had photographed, and videotaped and recorded all the milking equipment problems and had lined up a team of experts to testify on Mr. Jeff's behalf during the original litigation. Mr. Bryson used this information and all of his skills and persuasive abilities to convince the insurance company and the high-powered lawyers that they would spend too much money trying to defeat us in court. The insurance company settled the suit out of court the day before the trial was to begin. Mr. Jeff received a nice settlement after legal expenses. Ironically, it was the exact amount of compensation he had asked for before any lawyers got involved, almost a decade earlier.

Mr. Jeff is still dairying today and enjoying his role in food production with a herd twice as large and milk production two and a half times what it was when the original problems were shown to me. I am proud to call such an effective food producer a friend!

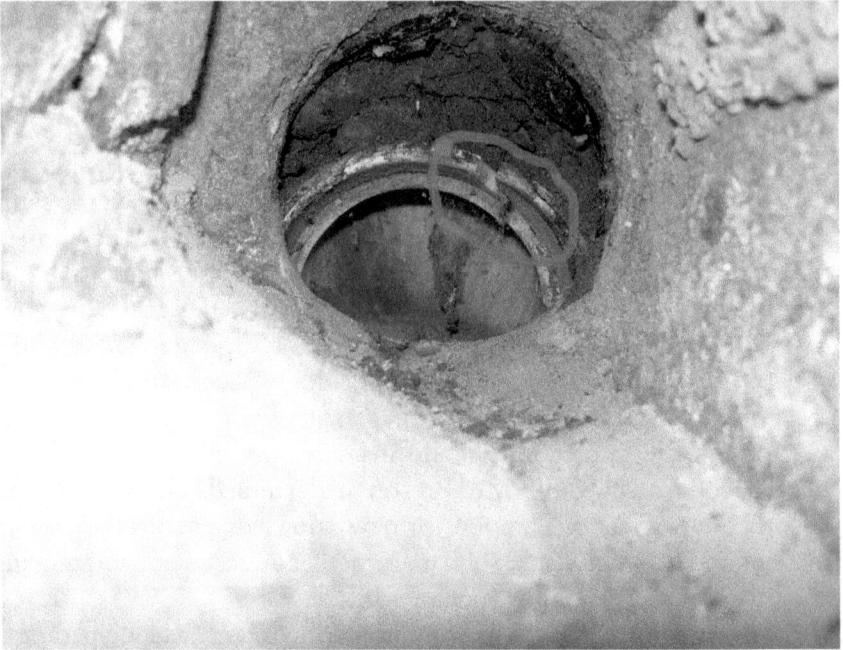

The red circle shows the location of the collapsed line which caused vacuum fluctuation and damaged the vacuum pump.

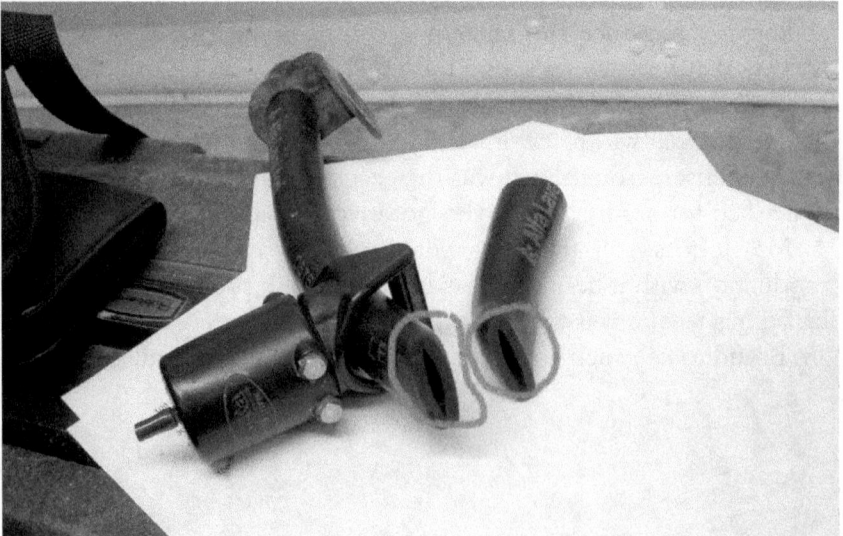

This photo shows the cheap pinch-type milk shutoff valve, which deformed the rubber milk line and restricted milk flow, causing vacuum instability at the teat end, which is a mechanical contributor to mastitis.

CHAPTER 21
Tennessee Farmers Coop Under Assault

I received a telephone request from an attorney in Knoxville, Tennessee late one afternoon. I was asked if I was willing and available to review some documents related to a case he was presently litigating between the Tennessee Farmers Coop and a farmer in east Tennessee. A majority of the litigations I have been involved in concerned me helping lawyers on behalf of farmers. This story is sort of different because I was about to help a farmer's cooperative, owned by farmers, defend itself from a lawsuit filed by a farmer.

For me, justice is justice no matter which side was wronged. I always reviewed the case records before I signed any work contract to try and assure that I work on the correct or just side of a dispute. In this instance, I was a little conflicted. I scheduled a visit to Knoxville the next week at eleven in the morning.

When I arrived at the attorney's office in Knoxville, I was motioned into the parking garage of what appeared to be the tallest building in the city. I rode the elevator to the upper third of the building and got out to a spectacular view of the city. An attendant met me and ushered me into a wood-paneled conference room that had an even better view of the city. While I waited for a few minutes, she brought me coffee and took a sandwich order for lunch. A few seconds later, she brought in a large box of peculiarly labeled papers and set them down at the opposite end of the large walnut conference table. Professionally framed University of Tennessee posters and autographed photos from several sports events adorned the walls. Man, I was impressed! This lawyer, I mean attorney, had to be special.

A tall, fit, gray-haired gentleman sharply dressed in a tailored suit entered the room and introduced himself as Mr. Manson. He shook my hand and apologized for his tardiness and we both smiled. Mr.

Manson gestured towards a chair and we both sat down ready to talk business. He began by thanking me for driving this long distance, and made sure that I had the address and case number for my billing purposes. I was beginning to like him already. I thanked him for his interest in me and asked what I could do for him. He explained that he represented Tennessee Farmer's Cooperative or TFC on behalf of their insurance company, Coop Mutual. The insurance company had recommended me as an expert in dairy industry matters after meeting me in a vitamin case in South Carolina, and had forwarded to him a copy of my resume.

Mr. Manson liked the fact that I was a veterinarian licensed in multiple states, that I specialized in cattle, that I had documented nutritional expertise, and that I personally managed my own dairies. He continued by explaining that he needed me to find holes or problems in the case at hand so he could defeat a predatory local attorney who had encouraged numerous farmers to file frivolous lawsuits against TFC. Most of the farmers this attorney recruited as clients were delinquent on paying their TFC accounts, and the coop was pressing them for payment.

The local attorney had convinced the farmers that a countersuit was a way to slow the collection process, but his real motive was to extort settlements of the countersuits from the liability insurer, Coop Mutual. Unfortunately, TFC had already settled two such suits without mounting a defense at all, so the local lawyer reasoned that TFC was easy pickings. The defendants, TFC and Coop Mutual needed my skills to help win this case and stop this predatory local attorney. Mr. Manson offered to let me familiarize myself with the details contained in the box of peculiarly labeled, subpoena-obtained records. They had prepared copies of everything for me to take back to my office if I decided to join them.

I spent about an hour reading the opposing lawyer's countersuit and reviewing some of the records in the box. Mr. Manson waited patiently while I studied the documents; both of us finishing sandwiches which the attendant brought to us. I was the center of attention and felt like I was sitting in the front of a courtroom with everyone waiting for me to speak. Eventually, I consumed enough of the subpoenaed data to feel confident that I was on the correct side of this litigation, and to feel confident that I could help TFC win the case.

I asked how much time I had to get an expert report together for him, and he stated three weeks. The first hearing was six weeks away. He needed at least as much time to prepare as I did, after he received the expert report. With this information in mind, I signed a contract and gathered things to take back to the more private setting in my home office.

The original suit by TFC was an account collection suit aimed at encouraging payment of a large unpaid feed bill accumulated by a dairy. The local lawyer's counter suit alleged that cows were sickened by the feed, so the farmer had the right to refuse payment for defective product. In addition, TFC was responsible for damages to his cows for which he demanded compensation. The counter suit described a period of disastrous "milk fever" events that injured and even killed some of the dairy's cows. He attached a list of affected cows and demanded payment for them along with zeroing out his open account balance.

The local lawyer had somehow found out what dollar amount of claims would trigger the intervention of the liability insurer to proceed to litigation. Knowing this figure, he kept the damages claims below the amount. Consequently, settlement decisions previously had been made by the local coop store which feared courtroom drama and publicity. They just used the insurance company's money to make the settlements. In their mind, why risk a trial? In the local lawyer's mind, he had an effective scheme going!

I began my discrediting of the counter-suit case by examining the specifics of the alleged injured cows. This dairy farm used a sophisticated record system created by a group in Raleigh, NC called the Dairy Herd Improvement Association (DHIA). Dairy management is very complicated and very record-dependent. I had assisted as a beta tester with this record system and even used it in my own herds. I was able to download the plaintiff herd database into my office computer and search the history on all the cows. This database history included breeding records, calving records, milk production records, and some health records. The dairy owner and his lawyer had identified 22 cows that they alleged were injured by the feed. The cows allegedly left the herd because they suffered what their veterinarian called "milk fever."

To simplify, "milk fever" is a layman's misnomer term for hypocalcemia (low blood calcium) and has previously been discussed in other chapters. It is a mineral imbalance problem that can occur at calving in adult cows. When I researched the 22 cows on the list I found that 14 of them were never diagnosed pregnant during their final lactation and were sold to slaughter without re-calving. Without a calving event, these cows would not have experienced "milk fever." Six additional cows on the list were pregnant but were sold in mid-lactation for mastitis or foot injuries according to the records. There were only two cows on the list which actually died at or near calving and there was no cause of death noted in the records. Therefore, the alleged damages claim was not valid according to their own records.

I phoned Mr. Manson, told him these facts, and started my work on the expert opinion letter detailing my findings. Faxed and mailed copies of the report were sent the following day. Mr. Manson was excited to get the report and scheduled a conference with the judge and the dairyman plaintiff's lawyer to request a dismissal of the suit. However, local judges in Tennessee are elected by the local populace and Mr. Manson did not vote in that district. In order to not offend the local dairymen voters, the judge denied Mr. Manson's dismissal request, and gave the counter-suit new life by allowing the plaintiffs to come up with an alternative list of cows. The plaintiffs quickly resubmitted another list of animals.

Mr. Manson apologetically sent me the new cow list. In all his years he had never seen a judge disregard protocols and act this way. I once again researched the animals on the new list. This time there were 20 animals on the list. To my surprise, all of the animals on the list were first-calf heifers, not cows. Heifers have different physiology than cows and don't experience "milk fever." In contrast to cows, heifers start out milking much less than adults and because of their rapid growth a heifer's enzyme systems are actively absorbing larger amounts of calcium from the diet than cows. Therefore, the physiology in heifers never allows blood calcium to get so low as to cause clinical "milk fever".

Once again, the alleged damage claims were not valid for the listed animals according to their own records. This information really excited Mr. Manson and he thanked me profusely. He realized that the local predatory lawyer had no one who could analyze the DHIA records. This time when he asked for another pretrial conference, he was prepared with legal precedents (prior judgements) that would discourage the local judge from denying his dismissal request. Denying the request would trigger a mistrial, a very embarrassing situation for a judge. The judge granted the dismissal and the local lawyer lost the case along with a piece of his reputation.

Nonetheless, this did not stop the predatory lawyer. He sued TFC at least three more times. I worked with another attorney to stop the local lawyer each of the three times he sued TFC. During the last suit attempt, he confessed to me that he was going to switch to human medical malpractice litigation. He felt there was more money to be made in that field. As I mentioned, I worked with a different attorney on the last three TFC cases. Mr. Manson was appointed to the Tennessee State Supreme Court shortly after our first collaboration. He really was somebody special!

CHAPTER 22
Sentinel Pigeons in Torviscosa, Italy

I made many visits to Italy for the Feruzzi Group over a period of 15 years. One of the primary stops was a dairy farm in Torviscosa, Italy. Torviscosa was a small town located near the Torvis dairy farm in the northeastern Friuli region of Italy. The Torvis farm was built long before World War II by Italy's infamous ruler Benito Mussolini, who was quite an agronomist. Mussolini created Torvis from a large marshy area by building pumping stations and canalizing the surface water to the pumping stations where the water was pumped out to the sea. He built several of these types of farms around the Italian coastline. I always enjoyed learning about Italy from my friend, Livio, manager of the US-based Open Grounds Farm. He typically set up these Italian farm visits and traveled with me. However, after his promotion to worldwide manager of farms for the Feruzzi Group he had other responsibilities when we traveled to Italy, and he often had to leave me on my own.

Torvis was a large farm of over 1,200 acres and there were numerous food crops grown on this farm in addition to the dairy production enterprise and a dairy foods processing plant. Even though I had worked at Torvis before (*Saving 300 Million*), every one of the early trips to Torvis began as usual with me touring the dairies and the farm facilities looking for opportunities to increase farm efficiencies. Late on one day I entered a feed storage area and noticed a large mound of soybeans in one corner of the barn. This mound had been accumulated during the harvest and cleaning of the soybeans for sale; as is required on the European open market. In the United States farmers are not required to do this cleaning before sale, so I asked what was to be done with the accumulated soybean cleanings, most of which were cracked or halved beans. They responded that they would be given to local farmers since they could not be used for animal feed. I was puzzled by this because I fed raw soybeans to cattle regularly in the United States without adverse effects.

The Italian farm managers had been taught that feeding uncooked or raw soybeans to any livestock was dangerous. It's true that soybeans contain a trypsin (stomach enzyme) inhibitor that can cause trouble in monogastric animals if not heat treated to inactivate it. However, cattle are ruminants and are not hurt by appropriate amounts of raw soybeans in their diet. I perceived an opportunity to change the diets of the dairy cows and save some feed costs.

Until this time, I had not been doing the nutritional work at the farm, and this gave me an opening to expand my services if I could cut costs and get the same or more milk production. That evening, I began the process of modifying my nutrition program to use Italian feed names, Italian costs, and metric weights. This process would take quite some time without Livio's help, but I needed something to do in the evenings on the multi-week long trips when Livio was otherwise occupied. I discovered that one could feel quite isolated by language and lack of transportation, so I tried to have projects to occupy my time.

Over multiple days I inspected the farm and observed the facilities and processes involved with making milk in Italy. I picked up a lot of vocabulary, especially in the area of nutrition and feeding. I gathered and translated many Italian farm-grown feed analysis reports and familiarized myself with locally available feed ingredients. By the end of the week I had completely adapted the nutrition program in my computer for use in Italy and had formulated a new feeding program for the farm. I was excited to share these feeding recommendations with the farm managers.

It was my usual mode of operation to have an end-of-visit exit interview or summary meeting which I later followed up with a detailed report translated into Italian. My friend, Dr. Livio, was usually in attendance for these meetings, but this time he was busy with the Feruzzi family in Rome. The farm manager, Dr. Prosperi, had a good understanding of English and this was very helpful. So, I made my presentation with the help of an interpreter and Dr. Prosperi. I was not aware of how important this presentation was to become. Livio was counting on good results to impress the family in his new role as worldwide manager. Dr. Prosperi was, however, a long-term competitive friend of Livio with a little jealousy over Livio's new success, and he was not ready to start taking directions from Livio and his American veterinary friend.

By using the whole, raw soybeans in the rations, I was able to save the farm 750 lire (75 cents) per cow per day in feed cost. The soybeans reduced the inclusion rate of two of the most expensive feeds, purchased soy meal, and purchased fat. It may seem that 75 cents per day savings doesn't amount to much, but when you feed 1,200 cows per day, that is a $900 daily savings, which equates to $28,000 per month and over $336,000 per year. In addition, I projected an increase in milk production of two liters per cow, which represented another $600 per day income on 1,200 cows. This production increase, if achieved, would yield another $220,000 per year for a total projected annual combined net profit of close to $600,000. After the oral presentation, I wrote the final report and forwarded it to Dr. Livio for translation into Italian. Livio was impressed with the work and the projections. I was pretty happy with it myself.

Then, weeks later, came the call from Dr. Livio, "What have you done? You have never been so wrong in 20 years of working with you! I have been ridiculed by the family for your recommendations to feed the whole raw soybeans to the dairy herd. How could you put me in this position?"

I was stunned! I was disappointed that my friend Livio was disappointed. What had happened in Italy? I asked for more information and Livio continued with the story. Dr. Prosperi told the family at a board meeting with Livio present that all of the animals to which he had fed the whole raw soybeans had died. He had not shared this with Livio before the meeting, so Livio had been caught completely by surprise and had no response. I asked what animal group had been fed the soybeans and how much soybean had been offered to the group? Livio then told me that Dr. Prosperi always double-checked feed recommendations from any consultant by feeding the product first to a group of pet pigeons he kept as sentinel animals. This is the first time that any of them had sickened and all of them died. He credited the pigeons for having saved the cattle herd from a disastrous fate. Livio then asked again, "What have you done?" Livio was livid!

I was surprised by this second assertion that I had done something disastrous; however, I knew that I had done nothing wrong in the ration. I calmed Livio down with the question of, "What will you do with the information about the real cause of death in the birds?" I explained that pigeons will quickly eat all the seeds they can hold at one time and store them in an anatomical structure called the crop located in their neck. They then later slowly process them for digestion. The trouble was that soybeans swell when they become wet, and this swelling of the wet seed caused the birds to suffocate. The pigeons had died of suffocation.

Livio proceeded to burst into laughter saying, "You ask what I'll do with the information? I'll have fun with this!" After Dr. Livio cleared his name and mine in this situation, the Torvis Dairy adopted my new feeding program with the raw soybeans, and became the highest-producing large dairy in Italy. The success of Torvis propelled our reputation in Italy to great heights and provided us with a foundation to build a new business—Worldwide Agriculture Consulting (WAC).

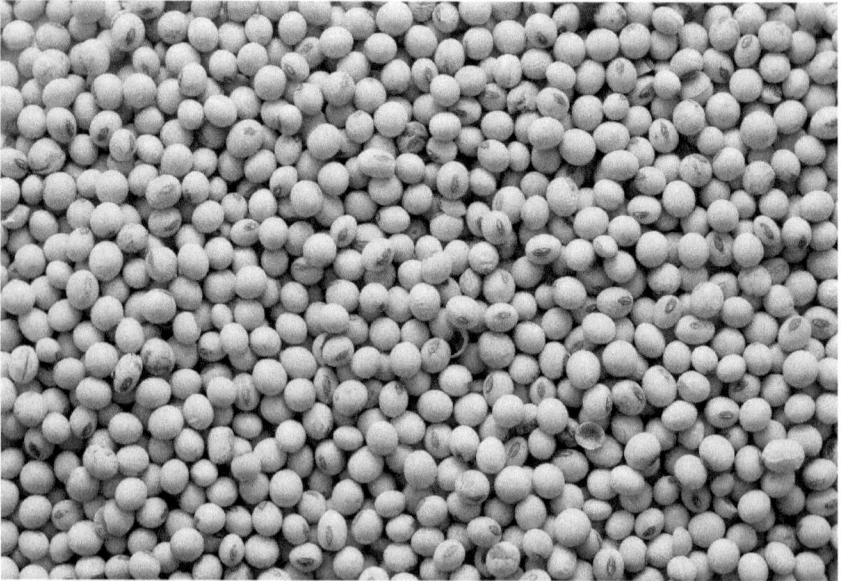

Whole Soybeans.

CHAPTER 23
Broken Bones in Le Galare, Italy

I received a telephone call late one afternoon from Dr. Livio, the worldwide manager of Feruzzi Group farms. He was calling from Italy to forewarn me that a new Italian farm manager was going to contact me about a problem occurring in bulls at the largest beef feedlot in Italy. The Feruzzi Group owned the feedlot. In this situation, I was not going to travel and investigate the problem. Instead, I was being asked to diagnose and resolve the problem by means of a telephone consultation only.

This was an unusual request for me at that time; however, now the majority of my consults are of this type. The call was to come the next morning in North Carolina which would be mid-afternoon in Italy due to a six-hour time zone difference. I had about twelve hours to prepare for the consult, so I began constructing a list of questions for history taking on the problem. I anticipated some difficulty collecting a good history because the questioning I needed to do with the farm manager would have to be asked and answered through an interpreter.

The call came as scheduled the next morning. The interpreter introduced himself in fine English and then introduced Dr. Pifinelli, the manager of Le Galare farm. After a few social niceties, we moved on to discussing the problem. I was told that the animals in the feedlot were all purchased as calves, and raised on bottles until they were old enough to be put on solid feed. Then, they were fed a ration made on the farm until they were sold for processing. Many of the calves were bought in France because they preferred the French Charolais breed. All of the calves were males, and they were kept in concrete-floored pens until they were sold. These procedures had not changed for decades, and they had had great success.

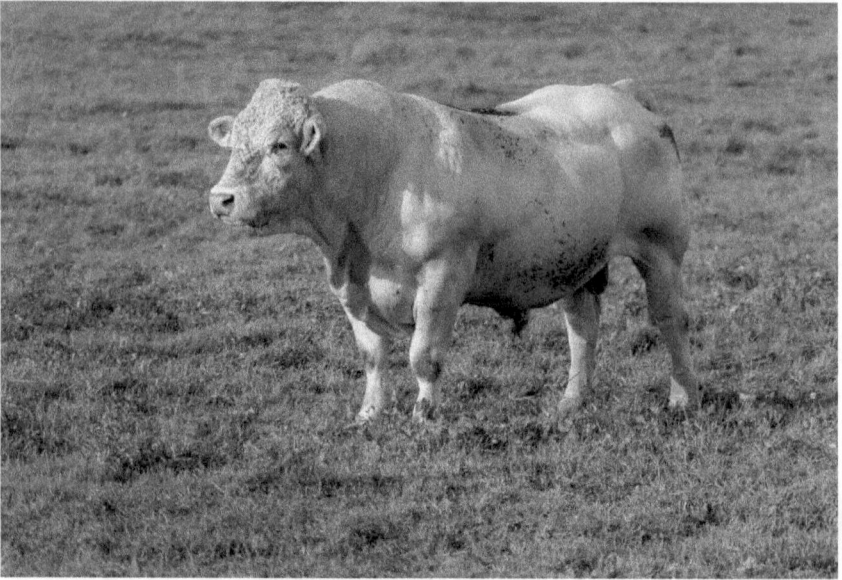

French Charolaise bull.

However, in only the last several months a third of the largest animals on feed were suffering random broken legs, just before going to sale. The animals were weighing about 1,500 pounds and of course could not be sold so they were destroyed. The farm veterinarian had taken blood from affected bulls and found nothing abnormal. X-rays of bones and analyses of bone samples were also made. Curiously, bone analyses were normal, but X-rays revealed thinning of the bones. The veterinarian could not explain the seemingly contrasting results. He suspected an infectious disease because nothing had been changed for years, but he did not know of any disease that could cause these symptoms. Dr. Pifinelli had been a friend of Dr. Livio for years, so he mentioned the problem to him, which led to this call. The farm had all blood, bone, and X-ray results copied and could mail them immediately.

Several things were remarkable from this history. The breed of the cattle, Charolaise, was a very large breed of over three thousand pounds mature weight for bulls, so they were powerful animals. (I was very familiar with the breed because my dad had started a herd of Charolais.) Also, these bulls were left intact or unsteered so they were reaching sexual maturity and experiencing testosterone aggression at about the time they were finishing up on feed. Both of these facts would predispose them to fights on the slippery concrete along with traumatic injuries. Nevertheless, these injuries had not occurred previously. The thinning of the bones on X-ray suggested a nutritional component to the problem, so I knew I needed to examine the ration.

I told them that I needed a copy of the ration, but they insisted on sending the laboratory work from the animals. I explained that the blood values and bone constituents were normal because the homeostatic mechanisms of the body closely regulated them. Therefore, those values would be the last things to change before death, and I didn't need to look at normal values. I suggested that the thinning of the bones indicated that there may be a problem with the ration; however, they insisted that the ration had not changed. I secretly began to question the assertion that nothing had changed and I gave them my contact information so they could send all the requested necessary documents.

In about a week, a package arrived from Le Galare. Inside were the X-rays, the normal blood samples, and the normal bone analyses. There was no copy of the ration. I thought my conversation had gone better than this! It was time to get in touch with my friend and mentor, Livio. In just another week a copy of the ration arrived. The problem for me was the entire document was in Italian. Livio was in Italy so he suggested I contact his nephew, Dr. Gabrielle, who was working at the Open Grounds Farm in North Carolina. I faxed a copy of the ration to Dr. Gabrielle and awaited his translation. He was able to translate all of the document except for one feed ingredient. Dr. Gabrielle apologized for not knowing the name of this feed, but it looked like it was a cement manufacturing residue.

I entered all of the feeds that were translated correctly into the nutritional program on my computer and back-calculated the ration. There were no problems with the ration I entered with these known feeds. So, I examined the unknown ingredient on the document more closely and realized that it was added at the bottom of the feed list using a different typewriter font. This unknown ingredient was the change in the ration I was looking for. The change in type font gave this American veterinary Sherlock Holmes the clue that broke the case. The farm manager, Dr. Pifinelli, had read an article written by a Texas feedlot that used cement kiln dust for a calcium source to save some minimal feed expenses. I had also read the article years earlier when it was originally published in a lay trade journal.

The problem at Le Galare occurred because the type of cement kiln residue added in Italy was high in phosphorus and was never analyzed before being added. This high phosphorus byproduct skewed or reversed the ration's calcium-to-phosphorus ratio. (If you wish for a better understanding of the underlying pathophysiology of this herd problem, a similar problem is described in Chapter 18, *Breaking Bones in Carolina*.) The incorrect calcium-to-phosphorus ratio caused the demineralization of the bones in the feedlot bulls.

My recommendation to Dr. Pifinelli and Dr. Livio was to remove the kiln dust ingredient from the ration. The problem of broken bones in Le Galare resolved quickly when this byproduct was removed. In later years, I personally visited Le Galare and met Dr. Pifinelli; and amazingly, there was never any acknowledgment that a change made to the original ration caused a costly herd nutrition disaster.

CHAPTER 24
"Assistenza Agricola" or Farm Assistance in Italy

After a few years of Doctor Livio and I working and consulting with dairies in Italy through our company Worldwide Agriculture Consulting, we were approached by a company named Cirio, Polenghi, de Rica (CPD). CPD was a large food conglomerate that produced and processed milk, pasta, and tomatoes. The company had seen the results of our work with a small number of their producers improving the quantity and quality of the milk which CPD was buying from them. CPD desired a contract with us for the purpose of establishing a farm assistance program that they would offer to all farmers that produced raw product for them.

This program was to be similar in function to the cooperative extension service in the United States. Doctor Livio would work with the agronomy (soils and plants) portion and I would work with the livestock (dairy) portion. For me, this work was both exciting and stressful. I knew the cows, the dairy business, cattle reproduction, nutrition, and diseases, but I didn't know the language and the people. Livio understood this well and spent a lot of time mentoring me.

CPD had great expectations for this farm assistance program which they titled "Assistenza Agricola." They expected the program to add value to farms by helping farmers produce more product and higher quality product. This improvement in farm profitability would allow the program to be used as a recruitment and retention tool for expanding the farmer base of their dairy food processing business. The growth of the raw product supplies would then fuel expansion of CPD's food processing business and fund the farm assistance service which would be offered at no cost to the farmers. The success of the whole venture was dependent on Worldwide Agriculture Consulting's ability to improve the quantity and quality of product sufficiently to attract farmers to CPD.

The program began with Livio and me visiting dairies all over southern Italy. We visited hundreds of small and large farms. We developed thorough checklists so farm evaluations would be comparable. We checked milk production records, milk quality records, cattle quality, milking system design, housing design, feed quality and quantity, and reproductive records. Where records did not exist we noted such. Where facilities were inadequate we noted this. Where cattle quality was poor we noted it. We pulled milk samples and feed samples for analysis.

Each farm we visited was thoroughly evaluated and the owner was interviewed to assess his willingness and ability to follow recommendations we would eventually make after the farm analysis was completed. Then before we departed the farms, almost all of the farmers would invite us into their homes for food, drink, and fellowship. They all had a relative or a friend somewhere in America! The Italian people are very gracious to Americans and showed us "Italian Hospitality."

As would be expected, the process was extremely time-consuming and tedious. Every other month I flew to Italy and worked for two to three weeks. The large amount of time I spent away from home put a strain on our family and would have been unbearable if not for my inclusion of the family in the travels. My wife made multiple trips and my children made multiple trips. My mother even enjoyed trips with us to Italy. The Italians were always welcoming. Doctor Livio and I evaluated the farms and eventually selected 65 dairies to begin the program.

I made written recommendations unique to each farm. Each of the dairies was enrolled for follow-up visits. During the process of following up with all the enrolled dairies, we elaborated a folder of Italian handout literature that had detailed instructions about reproductive procedures, breeding procedures, feeding program procedures, cow comfort and heat abatement procedures, milking procedures, calf raising procedures, and foot treatment procedures. Some of these procedures such as milking techniques were put on video tapes in Italian and shown during the follow-up visits. I wrote an Italian computer program that would balance the rations of farms based on the forage analyses we made in the United States.

In time I interviewed and hired a young Italian veterinarian and an

Italian farm technician who spoke fluent English to help with the follow-up process. We eventually set up a milk microbiology laboratory and a feed analysis laboratory to handle our quality control needs and reduce the cost of sample shipping.

Doctor Livio was soon able to leave me alone with the dairy program and develop his agronomy consulting with many of the tomato growers for CPD. For over ten years the "Assistenza Agricola" program was a remarkable success. CPD grew to handle over 35 percent of the milk produced in Italy. My records showed that we increased the average production of the dairies by just over ten liters of milk per cow per day. This is almost three gallons per cow per day over multiple thousands of cows! The success we achieved in this program allowed many farms to reach sustainability in continental Italy, Sardinia, Hungary, and Romania. Worldwide Agriculture's "Assistenza Agricola" program was also copied by many other consultants in Italy and in due course benefitted hundreds of farms and greatly increased food sustainability in Europe.

Even better, participation in this program was life changing for many individual dairy families. Several farmers who had never had the ability to do anything but stay at home to work became profitable, and they traveled to visit me in America where I was able to show them "Southern Hospitality." They visited in groups, requesting to see some good dairies and some beautiful places. So, I rented vans large enough to carry the whole group and traveled across North Carolina to some of my best client's farms on the way to beautiful state parks with waterfalls and gorgeous mountain vistas. Then, we turned east to end up on the Carolina coast with its large farms and beautiful beaches. Always included was a tour of the Italian owned Open Grounds Farm. The Italian farmers enjoyed the excursions so much that they reciprocated for me and my family later in Italy. I truly made a large number of friends across the ocean during my decades working in Europe.

CHAPTER 25
Ubiquitous Mycotoxins

I dealt with mycotoxins numerous times on various farms, so I felt that the best way to present some of these cases was to discuss them together. Mycotoxins are toxic metabolic products produced by molds (fungus and yeasts). Molds are everywhere in nature and are difficult to avoid. People have harnessed some good molds for flavor and preservation purposes in foods such as yogurt, cheese, and alcoholic beverages. These molds don't produce toxic byproducts if you consider alcohol nontoxic. Food animals are adversely affected by the mycotoxins of several genera of molds which attack grains and grasses.

Mycotoxins can vary in extent and type from year to year based on the crop growing conditions and the storage conditions. Mold spores need only moisture, warmth and a substrate (food) to grow. Most often there is no outward sign of the mold attack and farmers feed the produce to livestock only to realize later when problems arise that mycotoxins were present in the feedstuff. This was the situation in Chapter 10 (*Cotton Picking Changes*) which I presented separately because it resulted in a lawsuit. The following cases were similarly the result of unknowingly feeding mycotoxins in contaminated feeds, and they demonstrate several of the problems for which a practitioner should be on the alert.

***

I had just started working for an elite dairy farm named Kingsmill. The owner, David, had hired me to do some specialized reproductive work called embryo transfer. I had known David in another capacity for years and when he began looking for a certified embryo transfer practitioner he found me to be the one located nearest to his farm. For me it was an exciting opportunity to revive an old friendship and to work with some of the top cows in the Holstein breed. My first task was to super-ovulate and collect the fertile embryos from a cow he had just purchased for close to $300,000. She was the top show cow in the world when David bought her and her photo is shown in chapter 1 (*The Bomb in the Biosphere*).

He asked me to freeze some of her embryos and to transfer some of her embryos into recipient (surrogate) cows at another dairy farm. David told me that his partner had done some embryo work in the past and he would be available to help. David also asked me to help arrange the use of the recipient herd because he owned only a few cows at the time. I suggested the use of one of my client herds that I knew had a good reproductive history, and a deal was struck between the two of them.

The embryo transfer procedure requires that the recipient cows be at the same stage of the reproductive cycle as the valuable donor cow. I did the work of synchronizing the recipient cows with the schedule of the donor cow and then performed the collection of fertile embryos. After the embryos were evaluated and a portion frozen, David's partner and I drove to my client's farm to transfer the remaining fresh embryos into the synchronized recipients. The fresh transfer procedures went well with me transferring half and David's partner transferring half.

Driving back to David's farm we talked excitedly about the potential of the calves that would result from our work. About six weeks later I checked the recipient cows for pregnancy and found no pregnancies. What a tragedy! Those unique genetics were wasted. There appeared to be no explanation for the disaster until the milk plant called and gave the dairy a warning about high aflatoxin levels in the milk.

Milk aflatoxins come from the feed. I began testing the various feeds on my client's farm and found the commercial grain mix dangerously high in the mycotoxin, aflatoxin, from a mold named Aspergillus flavus. Milk levels above 20 parts per billion are a cause for discarding of milk, so my client quickly called the feed company and had them replace the contaminated grain mix with a clean mix. This solved the milk contamination problem and alleviated the nutritional stress on the cows, but the change was too late for the embryos.

Aflatoxin interferes with protein synthesis at the cellular level, and the rapidly growing young embryos were not able to cope with the slowing of their growth and died. Aflatoxins were the cause of the embryo transfer disaster.

***

Another client of mine, Mapleview Dairy, also experienced an aflatoxin problem. This client had invested in the equipment for processing and bottling their own milk, and for years had worked to grow a loyal local customer base. My family actually used their locally produced products. Mapleview Dairy was very diligent about getting their farm-produced milk tested by the state health department, just as is required of all other dairies in the state.

One month the state health department sent them a letter of warning about high aflatoxins in their milk. Knowing that the origin of the toxin was the feed, they sampled and tested all the feedstuffs on the farm. They found the feed corn which had been purchased from a local farmer was highly contaminated with aflatoxin. They immediately destroyed and replaced all of the feed corn because contaminated grain cannot re-enter the food chain. The milk aflatoxins disappeared.

Mapleview called me to ask what they should do with all of the milk they had placed on shelves in stores around the community. I recommended recalling all the milk to avoid the public's mistrust of their products. They decided to do the recall and also publish it in the local newspaper. We didn't know what this would do to the loyalty of their customers. Interestingly, after the milk recall their sales skyrocketed. People had never known of any other dairy processor that had recalled a product and felt that Mapleview Dairy was showing more care for customers than other milk companies. Afterward, the farm never bought feed corn which was untested for mycotoxins.

***

The Weathers Dairy in South Carolina was the largest dairy in the state for years. Readers were introduced to this farm in chapter 12 (*Please Pass the Salt.*) Being such a large size, a small decrease in the cost of feed would add up to a large savings. For this reason, they were always looking for and being offered deals on feedstuffs. I was there on the farm one summer pregnancy checking cows when I began to notice a significant number of reproductive record discrepancies. At this farm it was standard operating procedure to pregnancy check all cows bred for 30 days or more and not diagnosed pregnant, and to re-confirm pregnancies after 60 or more days pregnant. We would also recheck any cow that had been confirmed pregnant but showed signs of a repeat estrus event (heat).

During the pregnancy examinations, I was finding cows that were recorded as 35 days post-breeding to be 50 or more days pregnant. There were also quite a few re-confirmations of 60-day-plus pregnancies that were no longer pregnant, and there were numerous rechecks of cows that were 90 or more days pregnant that showed repeat heat signs. This scenario was unusual at the Weathers farm. Consequently, after the pregnancy testing was finished, I took the records to the office to speak with Mr. Weathers.

Too many pregnant cows were showing signs of estrus and estrus intervals were not normal in too many of the breeding animals. Mr. Weathers, who knew I was very accurate with staging pregnancies and respected my ability to recognize abnormal circumstances, responded by asking, "What could cause such a problem?" I suspected the presence of a feedstuff contaminated with the mycotoxin, zearalenone, produced by the Fusarium mold.

Zearalenone is usually more of a problem in swine, but it is known to have estrogenic activity in other mammals also. Questioning about recent purchases in the feeding program revealed that the farm had purchased some cottonseed at a bargain price. The cottonseed had gotten hot during storage and had spontaneously caught fire. The fire had been extinguished with water. This history revealed that warmth, moisture, and the substrate cottonseed were all present in the feed storage area concurrently.

I recommended that the cottonseed be removed from the ration immediately and I sampled the seed for testing. Laboratory analysis revealed that high levels of the mycotoxin, zearalenone, were indeed present in the seed. The remainder of the cotton-seeds were used for soil fertilizer and pregnancy checks returned to normal within a month.

***

Tall fescue grass is a plant of incredible importance to the beef industry. The grass was discovered naturally growing on a farm in Kentucky and after several years a university professor brought some of the seed to the University of Kentucky for propagation. When the university eventually released its Kentucky 31 fescue variety, it appeared to be the perfect grass for grazing beef cows.

It was adapted well to most of the Southeast and Midwest and Northwest parts of the United States. It stayed green long into the winter. It had a great nutrient profile for cattle and it withstood heavy grazing pressure. It is a perennial that thrives in heat and cold, so it would not need replanting year after year. It had drought tolerance and resisted insects. When cattle were not grazing, it would grow lush and tall enough to be cut for hay and it could be stockpiled in late fall for grazing in the winter months.

The "wonder grass" Kentucky 31 Tall Fescue, became so popular in the United States and abroad that more acres of it were planted than any other grass crop in the world — more than 35 million acres. It is one of the most important pasture species on the planet.

However, after the widespread adoption of KY-31 fescue, problems started to arise that eventually came to be known as "fescue toxicosis." It turned out that almost all of the seeds of KY-31 were infected with a fungus called an endophyte. This endophyte produced toxic ergot-like alkaloid chemicals which made the plant less desirable to eat. This endophyte lived symbiotically within the plant, and contributed to the hardiness of the plant by discouraging grazing and insect attack. As time went on the endophyte-infected grass would readily take over entire pastures because cattle selectively grazed other grasses and avoided the fescue. As grass stands became more dominantly fescue, symptoms of "fescue toxicosis" such as rough hair coat, weight loss, intolerance to heat, lameness, and poor fertility would escalate.

Eventually, the toxin in endophyte-infected fescue was discovered, and endophyte-free varieties were developed, prompting farmers to kill the stands of infected KY-31 and replant. However, the endophyte-containing grass was so much hardier that it quickly came back and outcompeted the endophyte-free varieties. Now, other varieties called novel endophyte-infected varieties have been developed. These varieties are infected with an endophyte fungus that does not produce the toxic ergot alkaloids. However, the novel endophyte still imparts some hardiness to the plants. The battle to replace the original KY-31 endophyte-infected grass on over 35 million acres still rages today, but we have more tools in our arsenal. A survey conducted in the year 2015 found that industry wide economic losses resulting from fescue toxicity has totaled over \$3.2 billion. Much of the losses were from reduced growth and reproduction.

The University of Kentucky now recommends the following:

> *Avoid grazing endophyte infected pastures during critical times. Don't graze high endophyte pastures just before calving and just before breeding. If possible, graze other species for around 60 days after calving. Also don't use infected fescue with lactating dairy cows.*

If farmers fully follow these instructions they will find that there is little opportunity for grazing infected fescue at any time during the year and in my opinion, it should never be used along with an embryo transfer program. Sometimes when things seem too good to be true, they are not true — "wonder grass or toxic curse."

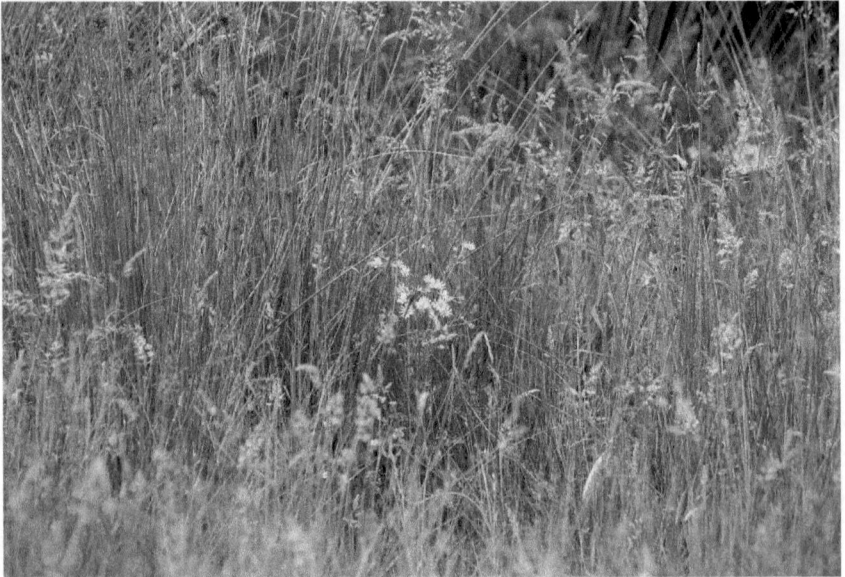

Fescue grass.

***

I am sure that advanced reproduction technologies are an important part of the solution for feeding the world. It is important for the developed world to share its genetic progress with the rest of the world's food animal farmers. This is being done today through artificial insemination and embryo transfer. In successful embryo transfer and artificial insemination programs it is essential to have the correct estrus synchrony between the recipient mother and the new germplasm used to make her pregnant; or, there will be no new successful pregnancy. Mycotoxins quite often interfere with the essential synchrony in these high technology reproductive processes.

At a client's farm in Virginia, I experienced an excellent example of this interference when I used hormones to synchronize a group of 25 dairy heifers to receive frozen embryos. Many of the heifers were observed to be in estrus (heat) before the hormones should have allowed them to be. Physiologically they should not have been able to show estrus with the synchronization hormone implants in place. After examining the heifers I concluded that some of them were still in estrus a week after the first signs of heat—much too long a duration of estrus. I suspected an unknown source of estrogen, perhaps the mycotoxin zearalenone. I eventually could use only four of the 25 heifers as recipients for embryos, when normally I should have used at least 20.

My Sherlock Holmes character emerged! In view of the synchronization failure, I took samples of the feedstuffs being fed to the heifer group before leaving the farm. Laboratory results revealed that the barley silage being fed contained high levels of zearalenone. The barley silage was being fed as the sole forage to the heifer group so it comprised a large percentage of their daily intake; however, the same silage was also being fed to the lactating cows at a lower inclusion rate. Probably all the animals receiving this feed were being adversely affected in their reproduction systems.

We eliminated the forage from the rations to improve reproduction in this herd. The farmer never suspected his forage was highly contaminated even though he remembered that he had difficulty with the harvest and storage of the crop. He had to add water on the feed as it was harvested to get it to properly pack in the silo and not get hot in storage. Apparently there were some "hot" spots in the silo anyway. There were warmth, moisture, and a substrate in the silo — the perfect environment for fusarium mold to produce zearalenone. Looking back, we were fortunate that we found the problem in the heifer group before reproduction efficiency was disastrously reduced in the lactating herd. Molds and mycotoxins are ubiquitous and insidious. Food supply veterinarians must be alert to the symptoms of their presence.

CHAPTER 26
Cows Can't Fly but Can Get High

In the winter in North Carolina, we always move back to Standard Time. In the Daylight Savings time of the year, we felt like we had time to get our work done before dark. This is not the situation in winter Standard Time. It gets dark at five o'clock in the evening. The early darkness can adversely affect one's powers of observation when examining a sick animal in a dimly lit dairy barn.

Such was the case one cold evening when I was returning from a distant herd check at about 5:30 and received a call from a favorite local client, Walter. He requested I see a cow right away that had been acting strangely all day by standing in a pond and refusing to get out. It took them all day to locate a cowboy with a horse to rope the cow and move her to the barn. Dairy cows don't act this way. I was curious enough to agree to the farmer's request, even though I was not on call that night.

When I arrived at the barn the cow was standing quietly in a pen. Walter had a halter on her tied loosely to a ring in the wall. I began my exam by putting a thermometer in her and while I waited for the temperature to register I began my patient history taking. There was not much history to take though, because this was a dry cow not due to calve for several weeks. She had not had any trouble in her previous lactation. She just decided to go for a swim on a cold day and not leave the pond until the horse pulled her out.

The physical exam did reveal some abnormalities. The temperature was mildly elevated a couple of degrees. The heart rate was rapid and no gut sounds were audible in the abdomen. I rectally examined the cow and found scant manure, but the calf was still there and alive. The rumen seemed to be mildly distended with gas. These symptoms pointed towards what could be a potentially serious problem of bowel blockage. These blockages do occur in cattle but they are rarely detected before the animal is too far gone to treat. I remember as a boy, my dad had a prize bull die from this. I explained my presumptive diagnosis and suggested that Walter load the cow on a trailer and take the animal to our clinic where we had everything we needed for abdominal surgery in a well-lit, clean surgery stall. Walter agreed that it was too cold and dark to do surgery at the farm.

Walter dropped the cow at the clinic and left her with my staff. I directed them to put her in the surgery stocks and start intravenous fluids immediately while I gathered materials for surgery. We hung up a five-gallon jug of fluids and started a fast drip—yes, in large cows we have to use these large volumes of fluids. During this time, the cow just stood quietly and stared out into space as if to be enduring pain. It took about an hour to gather the surgery materials, clip hair on the right side of the cow's abdomen, and aseptically scrub the surgery site.

When about half of the fluids were run, I noticed the cow looking more alert. She started to notice the crowd around her and follow people as they walked by. I decided to re-do the physical exam. The heart rate had returned to normal, and gut sounds were again present in the abdomen. The temperature had even returned to normal. It was now about eight o'clock, and the cow was no longer ill! I made the executive decision to put her out in a hospital stall and delay the surgery until the next morning if she was no longer normal. What a mystery!

The next morning I went in to the clinic early to examine the mystery cow. She was perfectly normal. I was delighted that she had recovered, but I could not explain to the farmer why she recovered. I called Walter and told him all the truth I knew and suggested he come pick up his normal cow. I then began my distant farm visits for the day.

Since I got an early start, I returned to the clinic early that afternoon while the sun was still shining. I checked to see if Walter had picked up his mystery cow and to my surprise, I found another different cow in the hospital stall from Walter's dairy. It was another dry cow that had been in the pond. The physical exam revealed a similar situation with a rapid heart rate, minimal gut sounds, and scant manure, but a live calf. This time there was plenty of light so when I checked the eyes I was surprised to see that the pupils were widely dilated. The cow last night also had dilated pupils but they should have been dilated when it is dark. Today the sun was shining directly into the eyes and the pupils should have been closed tightly. This cow was high on something! I suspected a toxic weed called Jimson Weed that contained an atropine-like alkaloid. Atropine is often used to dilate eyes for ophthalmic exams.

I called Walter, told him my suspicions, and asked if I could come over to walk his dry cow pasture. He, of course, agreed but jokingly said that there was no Jimson Weed around unless the cows could fly. I motored over and met Walter. He suggested that I ride in the back of his truck because the pasture was large. This sounded like a good idea since the sun was getting low. We rode the perimeter of the pasture and I spotted a broken down fence. The cattle had found a low spot in that old fence around an abandoned hog pen. There in the pen were several Jimson Weeds with the tops eaten off. Embarrassed, Walter admitted he had forgotten about that old hog pen.

I teased, "Cows can't fly, but they can get high!"

***

Over the years, I was called to numerous scenes of maladies caused by toxic plants. It was not always as much fun as this last story, but there was one more where I did get quite amused while solving it. It was down east in North Carolina at the farm of a rural high school teacher and his lovely family. The family did many things together and one of their favorite things was participating in rural agriculture clubs like 4-H. The dad's name was Denny and his teenage girls thoroughly enjoyed the competition of showing beef calves. Actually, I think Denny enjoyed the competition and the girls enjoyed working with the calves.

Denny questioned many of the show winners and determined that their edge was the genetics of their livestock. Most of them had been breeding cattle for years and had developed very good animals. To be competitive in a short time Denny would need to make genetic progress rapidly. He could not afford to buy the top Angus (solid black) calves, but he could afford very good frozen embryos. He just needed to find someone to help him get pregnancies with the frozen embryos.

Denny had not been in the livestock business very long so he asked around and found that I did the work he needed. He called me to his farm for a consultation on embryo transfer and to meet his daughters.

After about two hours, Denny and his girls were convinced that they could do their part in the process, and we made plans to get started. Only two things were lacking—the embryos and the recipients. Denny said he had located the embryos and would get them. I volunteered to locate some dairy heifers for recipients because they would give more milk and raise a bigger calf. Denny liked the sound of this! I found him eight breeding-age Holstein (black and white) heifers.

Denny and the girls liked to show in the fall calf show window from September through December, so we did the work in January in order that the calves would be born in early September. All this planning and scheming excited Denny and the girls. We synchronized the Holstein heifers and transferred 8 embryos. By the first of March the heifers were checked for pregnancy and five pregnancies were on the way. My work here was done or so I thought.

In early April I got a call on my cell phone from Denny. He was in a panic! Denny excitedly told me that his cattle had a terrible skin infection.

I asked, "Are all of the cattle affected or just the dairy heifers?"

He said, "Wait a minute. I'll go look." I held the phone until he came back to the phone and asked me, "How did you know it was only the Holsteins?"

I responded, "I didn't know. That's why I asked." Then I asked, "Is it only the white spots involved are both the white and black areas affected?"

Denny responded, "Hold on, I'll go look." After a few minutes, he asked, "How did you know it was only the white spots?"

I laughed and said, "I didn't know. That's why I asked. Could you go and look at the white areas of the bellies of the Holsteins and compare them to the white spots on the top of the back?"

Denny, out of breath, once again ran outside without saying anything. He came panting back to the phone and asked, "How did you know the bellies were okay?"

By this time I couldn't hold back and I chuckled over the phone, "Ha, ha, I didn't know. Ha, ha, ha, that's why I asked. Your cattle have been eating an early growing spring plant that has caused a condition called photosensitivity. It makes the unpigmented skin sensitive to direct sunlight and the white areas have no pigment. The white spots on top of the back will be the first areas affected by the direct sun."

Denny responded, "I knew there was a reason I liked Angus cows.

None of them are hurt. What can I do to the Holsteins?"

I laughed once again and said, "You can cover them with sunscreen, ha, ha, or keep them in the barn during the day and graze them at night until your native pasture gets bigger. They'll stop eating the other plant when the grass is available. Ha, ha."

This story has little to do with feeding the world but it was fun working with these fine people and their hobby. I lost touch with Denny over the years and don't know if he and his daughters ever won any trophies. My guess is they stayed with this livestock showing only as long as the girls were eligible and enjoyed it. The effort and funds required to raise livestock is considerable and it does not make a good hobby!

CHAPTER 27
Unable Germplasm in Virginia

Even though Southern Virginia is north of the Carolinas it still experienced the same summer heat and humidity as the Carolinas. The summer heat and humidity put a lot of stress on cattle, usually resulting in lower breeding rates and less need for pregnancy work in the summer. I always thought this was somewhat of a blessing for me because my children were out of school in the summer and I had a lighter work load, allowing me to spend more precious time with the family.

The cows under heat stress held that it was too hot and uncomfortable to show signs of estrus (breeding receptivity) and when they did show signs they were less fertile. In the southern heat, conception rates typically dropped below 15 percent, in contrast to above 50 percent in cooler weather. Nonetheless, for economic reasons, the farmers continued to try to impregnate cows in the summer and beat the odds against the process. The result was that there was always some nominal summer work for me to do. It was during a summer herd pregnancy check in Southern Virginia that I stumbled upon a unique problem.

Southern Virginia is a beautiful area. Rolling hills, rivers, and lakes abound. It was my joy to work in the area for many years. One of my favorite farms, Park Forest Farms, was located on the banks of the Roanoke River near South Hill, Virginia. The majority owner and also farm manager, Bill, lived on the farm in a restored antebellum home named Eureka, which was on the Virginia register of historic buildings. Bill's daughter married the Virginia Commissioner of Agriculture at Eureka in a lavish "Southern Era" wedding that my wife and I were invited to attend. I was honored to call this family both friends and clients for many years. Park Forest Farms was a fitting representation of both the past and future of southern agriculture. Operationally, it was an unsurpassed modern farm focused on high milk production and cutting-edge genetics.

Park Forest Farms was a member of a small bull proving syndicate called Virginia Genetics which produced and proved several young bulls each year for the commercial artificial breeding companies. Artificial insemination (AI) programs are where a breeding technician uses frozen semen to impregnate cows instead of natural bull breeding. To give more dairymen access to the best genetics, artificial breeding companies (bull studs) were established for collecting and distributing frozen semen to thousands of farms, instead of taking one bull around to a few farms. Almost all of the promising, high genetic young bulls have semen collected and frozen for use in programs designed to statistically prove a sire's value. If a young bull's statistical proof is high enough the commercial studs will buy him or contract him for distribution to the whole dairy industry worldwide. This can make the owner of the bull very wealthy.

Bill's experience in the bull-proving business allowed him to predict which young bulls would be the next leaders in the dairy industry. He was always using the newest, most promising young sires in the artificial breeding program at his dairy. He would use these young sires as soon as they were released onto the market, regardless of the time of year, so he did more breeding during the summer than most other herds. This required me to be at the farm monthly for routine checking of the cows.

With this background in mind, you can understand why Bill scheduled me to check pregnancies at the farm one hot August morning. We typically tried to finish by noon so that the cows would not be locked up in stanchions during the hottest part of the day. As the work progressed that morning I examined and treated recently calved cows for postpartum health, I rechecked older known pregnancies in valuable cows to verify that the fetuses were still healthy, and I examined cows with any new breedings over 30 days duration to identify the new pregnancies. Bill was present for the entire herd check recording the results of examinations on individual cow records. I began to worry about the new AI pregnancy results when we diagnosed only one positive pregnancy in the first twelve exams, so I brought this to Bill's attention. He chose to blame the results on the hot weather stating, "This happens every summer."

I reserved further comment until the herd check was finished. The final results were only one positive new pregnancy in eighteen breedings for a miserable five percent pregnancy rate. After I cleaned up I went looking for Bill. I asked Bill if I could examine the reproduction records for myself because the pregnancy pattern was not typical for his herd, summer or not. He led me to the office and gave me access to the records.

What I found reviewing the records confirmed my suspicions. Of the 18 breedings, 17 were to a "hot" new young sire called Lincoln. The only positive pregnancy was to the sole breeding of another older bull's germplasm. The new young sire's frozen semen had not resulted in any pregnancies. With my urging Bill sent a sample of this young sire's semen back with me to my clinic for detailed examination under a microscope. Actually, I also owned some of the same Lincoln semen at my small dairy back in North Carolina so I stopped by and picked up a sample from my farm, too, on the way to the clinic.

Both of these samples were examined under a high-quality veterinary microscope. I was befuddled when the semen showed excellent motility upon initially being thawed because I suspected maybe the semen had been mishandled while in transport to the farm by exposure to room temperature—a very common occurrence but not the situation this time.

On the contrary, after staining the individual sperm cells and examining them at 100 times their original size, the fertility problem was determined to be detached acrosomal caps. The acrosomal cap on the head of the sperm is necessary to provide enzymes used in penetrating the eggshell (zona) of the female's egg, thereby permitting the sperm to introduce its DNA into the egg to begin the new fetus's life. On all of these sperm cells the acrosomal cap was detached and did not allow the sperm to perform its vital DNA transfer function. Consequently, no new pregnancies or fetuses could be formed.

A little research revealed that a common cause of detached acrosomal caps is improper semen freezing technique. I looked up the telephone number of the commercial artificial breeding company and recorded the freeze code numbers printed on the straws of semen samples involved in the infertility problem. When I telephoned the bull stud, I was transferred to a technical services veterinarian who was very helpful. He related that the company always kept samples of all frozen semen that had been approved for shipment, and he would check the retained "house" sample.

(a) (b)

(c) (d)

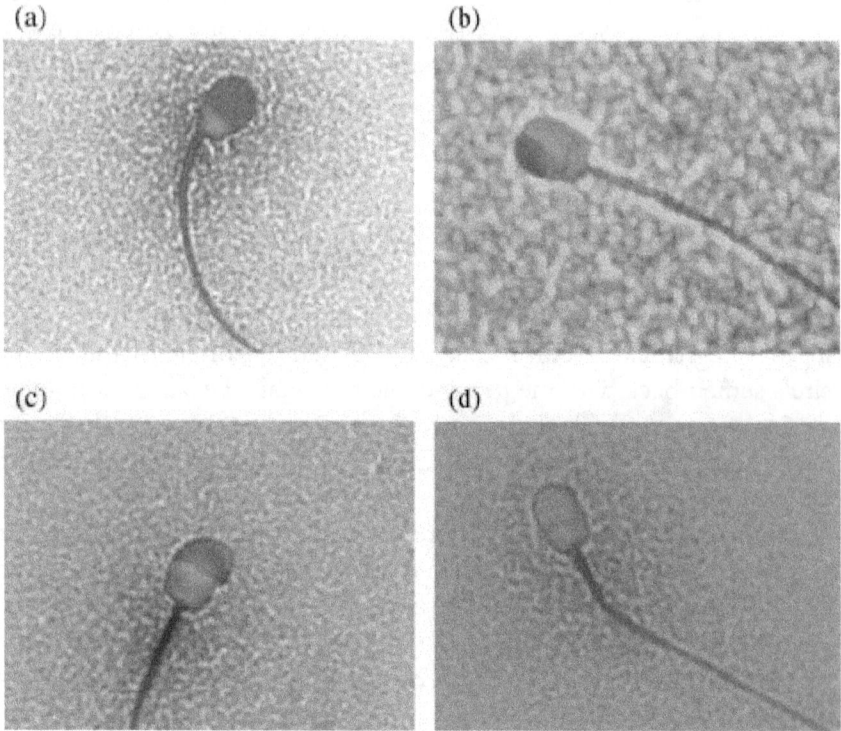

Acrosome intact sperm appear blue (a) whereas damaged acrosomes are evident by mottled or patchy staining (b) or a detached membrane (c). Sperm with a missing acrosome have a white or pink cap, with no blue staining evident (d).
Spindler, Rebecca & Huang, Yunren & Howard, J & Wang, P & Zhang, Hemin & Zhang, Guiquan & Wildt, D. (2004). Acrosomal integrity and capacitation are not influenced by sperm cryopreservation in the Giant Panda. Reproduction (Cambridge, England). 127. 547-56. 10.1530/rep.1.00034.

An hour later the technical services veterinarian called me back and thanked me for quickly identifying this problem and saving his company from some embarrassing conversations. He had already issued a worldwide recall and replacement on all of this Lincoln bull's improperly frozen semen. The potential economic damage from reproductive failure in the dairy industry could have been enormous.

This case of "Unable Germplasm in Virginia" became one of my favorite classroom examples of the fitting use of Sherlock Holmes's methodology of observing and then recognizing an abnormal occurrence or pattern at a dairy farm. Sherlock Holmes's techniques can surely have a place in the epidemiological investigations of food supply veterinary medicine problems.

CHAPTER 28
Uncharacteristic Rabies

If a veterinarian is fortunate enough to gain the trust of farmers, one of the benefits of doing food supply veterinary practice is the ability to participate in long-term relationships with farm families. Alvis was a dairyman I truly respected and enjoyed working with for decades at Sunny Acres Farm. He was an excellent businessman and cattleman and loved producing milk for a livelihood. He was also a man of strong faith who shared and acted on his faith. I was astounded when he generously supported me in my volunteer mission work around the globe. Alvis and I developed a close kind of relationship that is rare among men with such large age differences, for Alvis was 15 years my senior.

Alvis worked hard every day at his dairy and it pained me in later years to see father time take its toll on Alvis's health. Several years after two knee replacements and hearing loss he decided to sell out. I still remember the disappointment I felt the day he had me check his cows for the last time. Nonetheless, Alvis had a son named Charles who stayed on and continued to operate the farm with beef cattle instead of dairy cattle. Charles and I also developed a good relationship but the roles were somewhat reversed, as I was 15 years his senior. I became a trusted advisor to the next generation on Sunny Acres.

One late fall day I answered a telephone call from Charles at about nine in the morning. He usually treated common maladies in the herd himself but this day was bothered by the strange actions of a four-month-old calf. At four months of age, calves are self-sufficient but they still should stay close to their mothers and the herd. This calf was alone, separated from the herd, and far from Mom. The calf looked dazed or uninterested in its surroundings, was not eating, and had a wet muzzle as if it had been drooling.

Charles's question for me was, "What do you think is wrong with him?"

I had my usual response ready for Charles, "This is not enough information."

I asked if he had taken a temperature which is the most important basic signalment in a sick calf, and he responded negatively. He said, however, that it would be easy to catch the calf. I instructed him to catch, isolate, and get me some more information. I desired to know his temperature and wanted him to examine the mouth for any cuts or blisters. I also instructed him to use rubber gloves for his safety during the examination. I further questioned him about other animals, changes, and problems in the recent past. He shared that he had had a cow die the week before but thought little of it because she was very old. The only change he made was the source of purchased hay he was feeding about 10 days before.

The change to unknown hay preceding the herd problems immediately alarmed me. Much of the hay grown in his area contained higher amounts of a toxin called "nitrate" due to the excessive use of manure water irrigation on hay fields. I voiced this concern to Charles. He suggested that he could remove the new unknown hay from feeders and go back to the old hay he was feeding before the problems started.

He stated, "I'll examine the calf and move the hay, then call back within an hour."

I asked him to take a sample of the new hay for lab analysis when he moved it. He concurred and somewhat over an hour later called back with the requested information on the sick calf, but there were more problems. When he was moving the hay he observed a cow separated from the herd and she came up near the tractor, acting wobbly. He continued that before he could finish moving all the hay she stumbled away and fell over dead. He was distraught!

I calmed him down and returned to the history taking. The temperature on the calf had been subnormal, not unusual for a calf not eating, I thought aloud. There had been only slight abrasions in the calf's mouth, possibly from the rough hay. That could explain the drool around the mouth. Charles and his herdsman had used gloves as instructed to examine the calf. Charles asked for more guidance. I instructed him to load the recently deceased cow on a trailer and transport it and the hay sample to the North Carolina State Diagnostic

Laboratory in Raleigh, North Carolina. Charles agreed and anxiously got right on it. It took about two hours to get to the lab. I called ahead to direct the lab in its diagnostic efforts.

Later that same afternoon the lab called me with negative results on nitrate tests in the cow so my number one etiology (cause) was lowered on my list of causes. I began to suspect exposure to some other toxin such as poisonous plants. I then telephoned Charles to give him the new information and share my new suspicions. I asked him to drive the perimeter of his pasture and look for any poisonous plants such as wild cherry trees, pigweed, or jimson weed which could have been eaten by his cattle. Charles countered that he didn't know any of those plants. I suggested he telephone his local Cooperative Extension Service and get their help.

Within minutes Charles telephoned me back and relayed that the extension agent said he was unable to travel to Sunny Acres until the next week. I felt the situation was too critical to leave unsolved, so we agreed that I'd drive up early the following morning. So, the next morning I gathered up my plant books and headed north to Sunny Acres.

While in route, I telephoned the feed analysis lab for any results from the hay sample and found that the hay was similarly negative for nitrates. Charles telephoned as well while I was in route to his farm and excitedly communicated that there was another older calf acting disoriented this morning and that the previous day's sick calf had died during the night. Things had gotten considerably worse at the farm! Then just before I arrived at Sunny Acres I received another telephone call — this one from the state diagnostic lab. The autopsied cow's brain was positive for rabies.

I had asked the lab to test for this disease since I could not rule it out based on symptomatology, and I knew that Charles and his hired help were going to handle an affected calf. In over 40 years of specializing in cattle veterinary practice, this was the first time I had encountered rabies in a cow!

During my military service in the United States Air Force I had been the rabies control officer on my base, so I had studied rabies thoroughly. Rabies is a virtually 100 percent fatal viral disease of the nervous system. After a bite from an infected animal, the virus infects nerves near the wound. The rabies virus then travels, protected from the immune system, through nerve fibers from this wound to the brain where it causes a lethal disease. Most spread of rabies is typically caused by a carnivore. Carnivores (meat eaters) like cats, dogs, raccoons, skunks, coyotes and bobcats etc. experience a "furious" form of rabies just before they die which makes them dangerously aggressive. Cattle and most other herbivores (plant eaters) experience a "dumb" form of rabies that makes them act disoriented. Rabies is therefore more difficult to diagnose in herbivores. Nonetheless, the saliva of affected animals is infectious in both carnivores and herbivores.

Rabies paralyzes the muscles of the throat, creating trouble swallowing and giving the affected animal the characteristic appearance of drooling or foaming at the mouth. The organ of choice for laboratory diagnosis is the brain. This is a dangerous disease and much effort is made to vaccinate carnivores against infection. However, little emphasis is generally placed on vaccination of herbivores because it is rare for them to pass the virus. That is except when someone purposely exposes themselves to the saliva as in Charles's examining of an animal's mouth.

Charles met me at the farm gate as I turned into his drive. We went over to the pasture where the disoriented calf was stumbling around and observed it for a few minutes. It was apparent that the calf had an old wound on its side, so I surmised this calf had rabies from an animal attack. We shot the suffering calf dead, through the heart, to not damage the brain and destroy the ability to test for rabies. A photo of the calf's wound is attached below. I removed the head of the calf for rabies testing before we buried the body. We also removed the head of the younger calf that died the evening before.

Just to be certain there were no toxic plants responsible for any of the deaths, we made a sweep around the pasture perimeter for toxic plants. No toxic plants were observed. Rabies was judged the cause of all the deaths and, fortuitously, it had been diagnosed within 24 hours of the initial telephone call!

While I was at the farm I discussed the danger of rabies with Charles, especially in light of his examination of the mouth of the first calf. I commended him for following instructions and using gloves in the exam, and I instructed him to call his physician to discuss post-rabies exposure treatment. Eventually, both Charles and his herdsman were given the post-exposure rabies treatment. The county health department was notified and stepped up to perform rabies vaccinations in all domestic animals on the farm and in the area, including dogs, cats, and horses. Below is the photo of the healing wound on the side of the suffering calf that was humanely sacrificed for brain rabies testing.

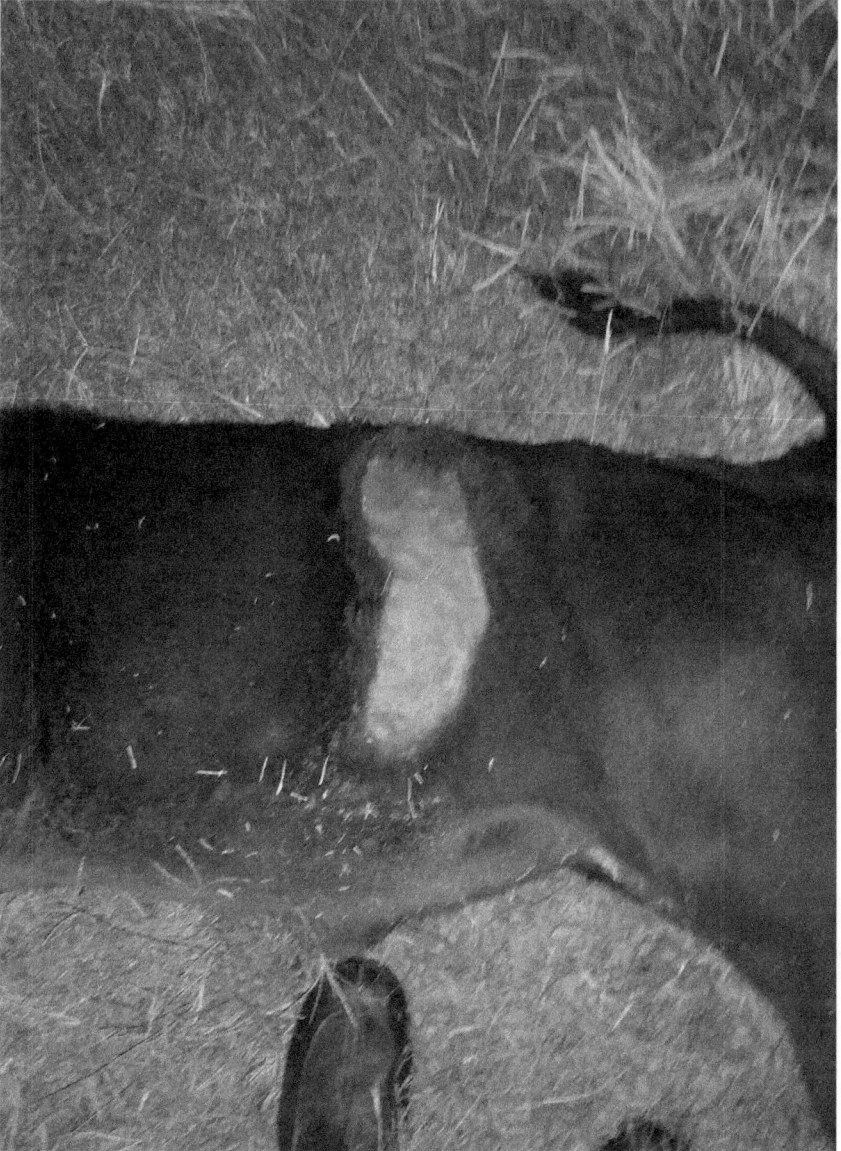

As I was leaving Sunny Acres, the North Carolina Area State Veterinarian arrived in official capacity to place the farm under quarantine for six months. This meant no cattle could be sold or brought in for the duration. The state veterinarian offered to take the two heads to the lab, so I transferred custody. The state would now finish the job of containing the rabies and preventing spread.

I thought my work was done until Charles asked me for further help. Charles typically sold cattle before the winter feeding period because he had limited hay and his pastures didn't grow in the winter. He needed help sourcing hay and feed for the extra cows he was required to keep on the farm until the six month quarantine was lifted. Charles didn't have the contacts necessary to find that unusually large amount hay.

Over the next weeks I helped Charles source feed from other clients of mine, and eventually enough hay was found to get him through the tough winter. In all, eight cows and calves succumbed to rabies at Sunny Acres in a short week or ten day period. The literature states that it is very rare for more than one or two cattle to die from a herd rabies event. This was a very unusual exposure with eight or more animals being bitten in a short time span. How many rabid carnivores came through the pasture at Sunny Acres? No positive carnivore was ever caught or identified, and now, years have now passed with no recurrence. Strangely uncharacteristic!

CHAPTER 29
The Belligerent Longhorn

I have always felt it important to support youth aspiring to get involved with livestock agriculture. Industry advocacy is what I like to call this important role of the food supply veterinarian. There is probably no better, nor more visible place to show this support than at the state fairs that are held around the country in the fall. This is the reason I annually volunteered to provide veterinary care at the North Carolina State Fair for decades.

My services usually were not needed until day three to four past fair opening day, after the animals had time to react to the changes in feed, environment, rest cycles, and pen mates. However, one year I received a telephone call from a Department of Agriculture veterinarian at nine in the morning before the noontime fair grand opening. She was frantically needing me to come to the fairgrounds to deal with a Texas Longhorn display cow that was acting aggressively toward the fair staff. She explained that the cow had calved the night before, and also had ugly afterbirth hanging down from her rear end. The government veterinarian had no drugs or equipment or even the experience to deal with the situation. This needed to be resolved before the fair opened and fair visitors were exposed to the offensive conditions.

At the time of the call. I was already deeply into my day's work of embryo transfer. I had already harvested twelve embryos from a superior donor cow and was washing them under the microscope for evaluation and grading. The embryos are actually live little calves seven days old, and their requirements to remain alive mandated that they be placed into a nurturing uterus as soon as possible.

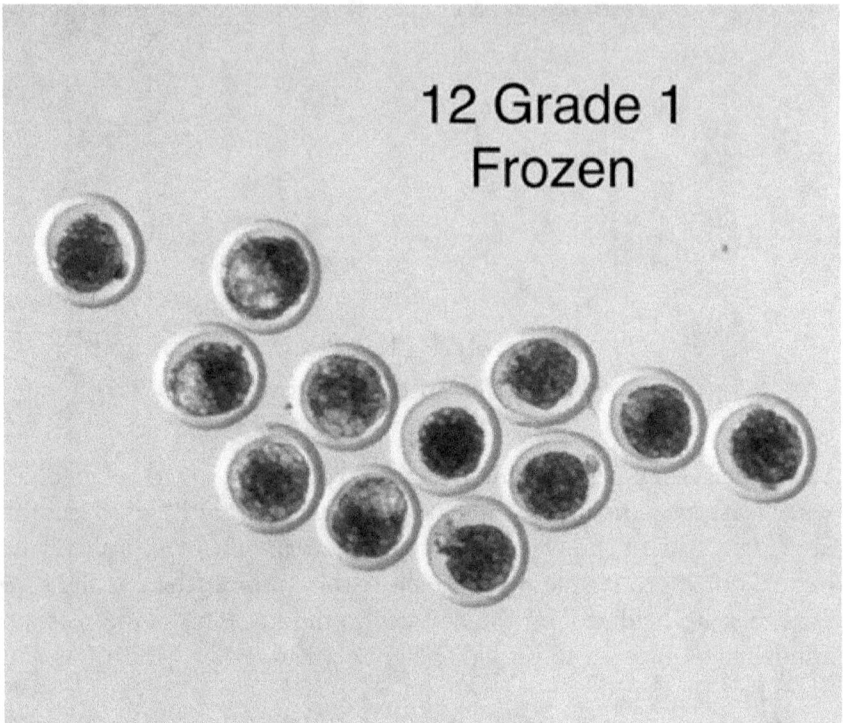

12 Grade 1
Frozen

This meant that I had to finish the work of transferring the embryos to recipient heifers, before I could attend to the state fair public relations calamity. I gently explained all of this to the state veterinarian and she countered that her alternative was to call the veterinary college which was just across the street from the fairgrounds. I encouraged her to call them if she could not wait for me. Nevertheless, she reluctantly made the decision to accept my projected timeline of a one o'clock pm arrival at the fairgrounds, only an hour after the opening.

Upon arrival at the back door of the main agricultural display building I was met by the state employed veterinarian. I gathered a bucket of soapy water, an obstetric glove, and a few pharmaceuticals from my truck. The state veterinarian quickly escorted me to the pen of the belligerent Texas Longhorn.

I stood and observed for a moment. The pen was a 15 foot square enclosure made of pipe gates locked together. The spacing between the pipes was about 12 inches, and the cow was busy holding a fairly large crowd of anxious fair staffers at bay by thrusting one of her four-foot-long horns through the pipes in the direction of the gawking bystanders. It was quite comical watching the diminutive 800 pound brown cow control the crowd. I thought of her as diminutive because she was small for a cow. I was typically handling full-grown black and white 1,500 pound Holstein cows.

The Longhorn's healthy calf, only a few hours old, was lying behind her in the clean, loose straw, admiring the bravado of its mother. The mother longhorn was periodically glancing at her newborn, not to see if it was watching her, but to ensure that it was still safe from the crowd of perceived human predators. Just as described by the state veterinarian, the cow's afterbirth had not dropped from her rear parts and hung in an unsightly manner all the way to the pen floor. It bloodied her legs and was gathering straw. In consideration of the whole picture in front of me, it was very difficult not to fall to the floor rolling in laughter.

I recouped my composure and asked the fair staffers to place a large tarpaulin over the pipe gate to obscure the fair visitors' views of the coming events. I then jumped into action. Literally, I jumped into the pen with the little brown cow and grabbed the far end of her right longhorn. I knew the little cow could do little to me with that four-foot-long horn lever securely in my hands. The bystanders were astounded enough to gasp! I then pointed to the two heaviest fair staffers in the crowd and called them into the pen with me. They were given instructions to each hold an end of the 8-foot-wide horn rack of the little cow, while I moved to the rear to take care of the mess back there.

I put on my glove, scrubbed up the cow's rear end, and removed the dangling afterbirth. After using the remaining soap to clean the cow, I gave her a quick injection to prevent infection. I then gathered the afterbirth into the bucket and climbed back over the pipe gate to safety. The two large gentlemen holding the horns looked anxiously toward me and I told them to simultaneously let the animal loose at my count of three and scramble over the closest gate. One, two, three, and everyone was again safe on the outside of the enclosure.

The "Belligerent Longhorn" sagely turned to attend to her calf. She smelled her precious, beautiful baby and realized that the humans had not touched it. Satisfied that she and her calf could be safe in this situation the little longhorn abandoned her task of intimidating the humans and quietly laid down in the straw to enjoy her new family member.

The state veterinarian shared with me that she had questioned her decision to wait four hours for me to get to the fair, instead of calling the veterinary college. However, in the past, when the vet school had come they made such a frightening display. They had anesthetic darted an animal and taken such a long time delivering the services that the activity really upset the fair patrons. She felt vindicated now about the decision to wait and she voiced her approval, because she really appreciated the calmness and quickness that an "old practitioner" was able to bring to the situation. The "Belligerent Longhorn" also showed her approval by humbly lying down with her calf as if nothing was amiss.

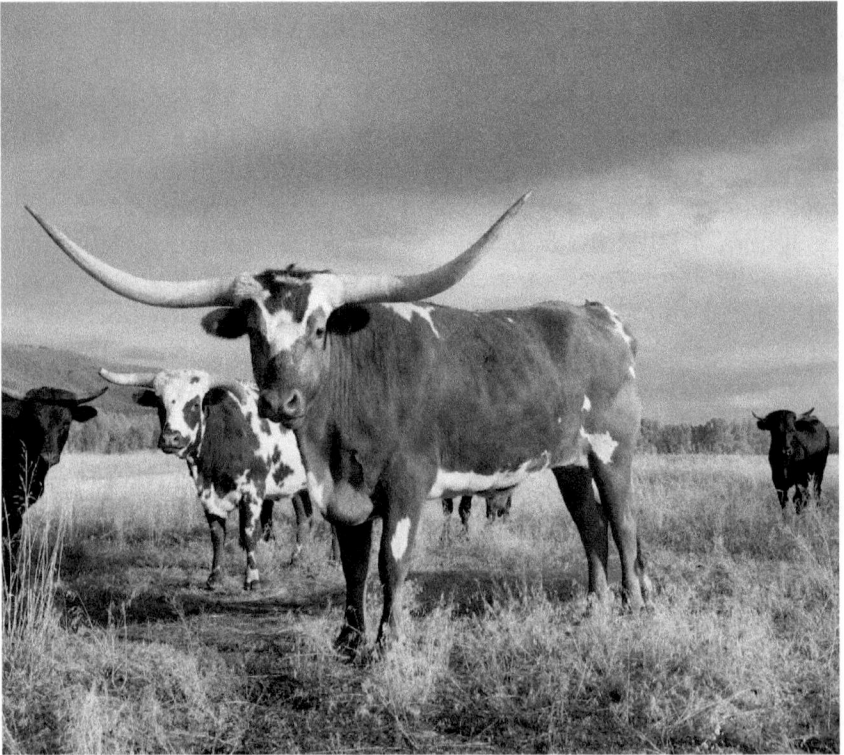

CHAPTER 30
Multiplying Pregnancies in Sardinia

A few months ago, I received a telephone call from Sardinia, Italy. It was Dr. Gabriele, the nephew of Dr. Livio, my past partner in the Worldwide Agriculture Consultants business. Gabrielle had been visiting his family in Italy when a worker at his brother's house mistook him for Uncle Livio. Gabriele and I have enjoyed a friendship for over 30 years, and he wanted to share the worker's story with me.

The worker had been formerly employed on one of our Italian dairy client's farms and he remembered both Livio and me visiting the dairy. Although it had been over two decades since we were there, he still remembered that we corrected a breeding problem at the farm.

Sardinia, Italy, is an island in a temperate climate zone, but it has an arid, hot microclimate. I did not realize how desert-like it was until I first traveled to Sardinia and saw the ancient Roman salt lagoons along the seashore. The Romans dried sea water in these lagoons for centuries to make salt from the sea. The hot, arid microclimate made this possible.

It was in midsummer when we visited Azienda Medda (the Medda farm) to investigate a breeding problem at their large 1,200 animal dairy. Cow conception rates, measured by pregnancies per breeding, were found to be less than ten percent during this sizzling time of the year. Although the owners accepted the low rates as normal during the hot months, I thought there might be another explanation because I dealt with hot weather in North Carolina every year, and our conception rates were not that low.

I began the problem investigation by reviewing records. By this time I was able to read and understand the Italian records fairly well. My review revealed that the dairy was artificially breeding exclusively, and it was using high genetic semen imported from Canada and the United

States. I used these same semen sources in the United States and knew them to be of high potency and quality. To save money, the herdsman would often breed two cows with one straw of frozen semen. I did this often at my farm in the States also, and it worked pretty well. I next examined the vaccination program and found it to be satisfactory. The most noteworthy detail revealed in the record review was that the conception rate was never very good, even in the cooler times of the year. This fact tended to validate my suspicions that there was more to the problem than just the weather.

I continued my investigation by rechecking for pregnancy all the cows that were bred in the past four months. I wanted to confirm that the local veterinarian was correctly diagnosing all of the pregnancies and that the records were accurate. I checked about 200 cows and heifers and found the records were indeed accurate. This palpation (manual feeling) work also confirmed that all of the cows had normal reproductive tracts and were ready to become pregnant. No cause for low conception had been detected at this point, so the investigation moved to observing the actual artificial breeding process.

During the palpation of the cows that morning I had found three animals that were in standing heat and were ready to be bred. We brought these cows into the breeding area. I intended to observe how the herdsman handled the semen and placed it into the waiting animals. The proper way to prepare the frozen semen for breeding is this: first set up a warm water bath at 95 degrees Fahrenheit, then remove the straw of frozen semen from the liquid nitrogen storage tank using forceps and quickly place it into the thaw bath for a 20-second thaw. Lastly the straw is removed from the thaw bath, dried, the tip cut off, and it is then placed into a warmed breeding gun for use.

Holy cow! I was shocked by how incorrectly the semen was being handled. The straw of frozen semen was picked out of the liquid nitrogen storage tank by fingers and held horizontally in the bare hand until it was cut in half by scissors. The half not to be used was placed back into the storage tank. The other half straw was thawed by cupping in the hands for a minute or so and was then loaded into a breeding gun for use.

Wow! In my assessment, the entire semen straw had been thawed in the warm hand and hot air before it was cut in half. Therefore, the half put back into the tank was killed by refreezing at incorrect temperatures. The half that was loaded into the gun was rendered subfertile by thawing at the incorrect temperature and being held for an extended time. It was no surprise that conception was low. The amazement was that there were any pregnancies at all.

I demonstrated the correct thawing and handling technique. I furthermore demonstrated how to breed two cows with one straw by correctly thawing and loading one whole straw into the breeding gun and expelling half of the semen into each of the waiting cows. The changes in the breeding technique resulted in a quadrupling of the conception rate in mid-summer. The Medda's were astounded by the results. They became some of our best clients and closest friends in Italy for many years.

Sardinia has the largest concentration of dairies in all of Italy. The word of our fertility success in the summer got out all around Sardinia and created a huge demand for our expertise. We could not get to all the work that came our way!

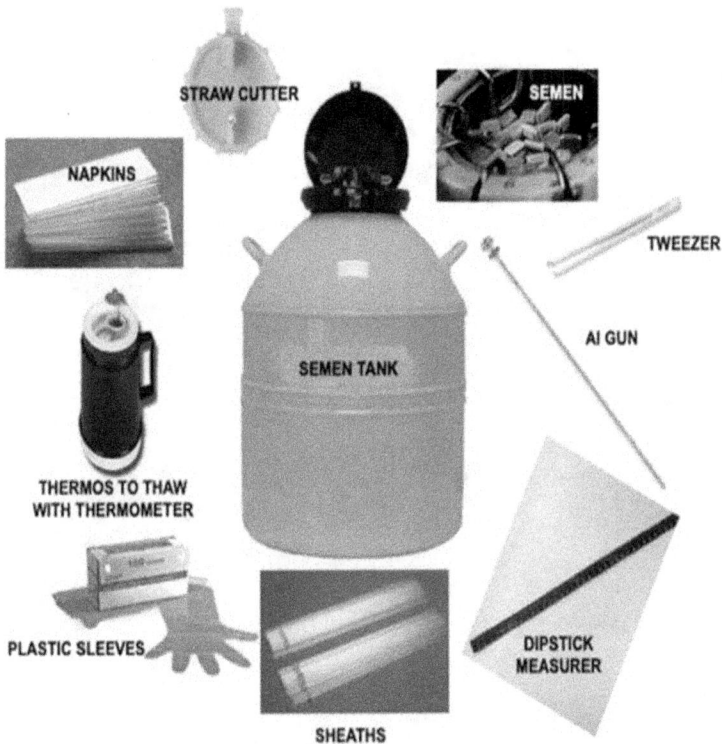

Basic equipment and material used for artificial insemination. Garcia Buitrago, Jose. (2021). Teaching Notes on Dairy Production. Reproductive Management of Dairy cattle. Artificial Insemination.

CHAPTER 31
Fertilizing the Cows

Over the 50 years that I have been involved with veterinary medicine there have been many innovations that have improved food animal practice delivery. The one thing that has had the most impact on my practice life is the cellular telephone. Cell phones permit immediate communication with clients at any time of day. This convenience allowed me to make callbacks to clients while traveling and untethered my practice from the home telephone. Cell phones turned my practice vehicle into an office on wheels and allowed me to spend more time with my family when I arrived home.

I received a cell phone call one day about noon while returning from herd visits in the western part of North Carolina. The call showed up on my phone as Barry, a man who worked for Earnest, a special client/friend of mine in eastern North Carolina. I assumed there was a problem at Earnest's farm, but as the conversation evolved Barry revealed a problem in his own cows. Barry was quite an entrepreneur. He worked for one cattle farm while hiring someone else to tend the cattle that he owned.

Barry told me that his employee had called him and reported the sudden death of three cows that were normal the afternoon before. Barry was headed to his farm and wanted me to come meet him. I explained that I was hundreds of miles from him and could not be there until the next day. He then asked me how we should proceed. I responded that cell phone conversations would allow us to begin the herd death loss investigation as we both traveled. I entered my Sherlock Holmes investigative posture and began a methodical history taking. The conversation went like this:

Doc: How old are the deceased cows? Certain diseases

have a tendency to strike younger or older animals.

Barry: All deaths were in middle age adults.

Doc: Have you added cows to the herd recently? A source of new disease.

Barry: not for years. It is a closed herd.

Doc: Do all the cows have calves at their side?

Barry: Yes.

Doc: Have you changed pastures or water sources recently? It could be related to something in a new location.

Barry: Not in years. It is a rented pasture.

Doc: Have you cleared or cut trees down along fences recently? Wilted wild cherry trees are extremely toxic.

Barry: Nothing in or along the pasture boundaries have been disturbed for months.

Doc: What type of pasture are they grazing? Some grasses and forages can pose risks at various times of the year.

Barry: They graze mixed, native pasture grasses, mostly fescue. Have been grazing these for years with no problems.

Doc: Are you supplementing any other feeds into the diet? A contaminated feedstuff could be a source of a problem.

Barry: This time of year we have never needed to supplement because grass is plentiful.

Doc: Are the cows on a salt and mineral program?

Deficiencies or excesses of minerals could lead to cattle eating abnormal things, a condition called pica.

Barry: My cows are on the same mineral program that you set up for Mr. Ernest's cows. Never had any problems in the past and mineral has not run out.

Doc: Have you worked or treated the cows in any way recently?

Barry: Not done this for several months.

Doc: Have you treated the pasture or fertilized the pasture recently?

Barry: I have not treated the pasture, but fertilizer was spread two days ago by a local fertilizer company. Mr. Ernest and I got a good deal on some fertilizer.

Barry answered all the questions as accurately as possible while driving to his cattle farm. He told me he would call back in a short time after he had time to see the situation at the farm.

The most implicating answer that Barry gave was that the pasture had been fertilized two days prior to the deaths. While I waited for his return call, I mentally ran through the ways to reliably diagnose if the cows were exposed to the toxic levels of nitrates which are present in fertilizers. When Barry called, he explained that the dead cows were scattered in different locations. They were fat, healthy cows with big baby calves. No signs of trauma or injury. I asked him additional questions.

Doc: Were the cows on the pasture when you fertilized it? If not, how soon did you return the cows to the pasture where they died?

Barry: The cows were on the pasture when the company spread the fertilizer. I have always done it this way.

Doc: Did you use liquid or granular fertilizer? Could

any of the fertilizer have gotten into the water or feed sources?

Barry: I am unsure of this, since I was not here when the fertilizer was spread. Water should have been safe because cows use waterers with fresh well water.

Doc: Were any other cows affected?

Barry: There were two other cows off away from the herd that looked disoriented and were breathing very hard and fast. Do you think they have it?

Doc: These two cows sound like they could be affected. Do you have a spare pasture you can move the cows to, if the herd needs to be removed from this pasture?

Barry: I can move them across the road into another pasture if necessary.

Doc: Did you take time to walk around the pasture to see if there were any accidental spills of fertilizer?

Barry: Not aware of any spills, but I wasn't thinking about this when I looked over the herd. I will go back out and look for this. I'll call you back in a few more minutes.

Doc: That is a good plan because, until now, there has been little to no highway traffic. But now as I approach a large city, I need to sign off for about 30 minutes.

Even though I was using the cell phone hands-free, I needed to focus more on traffic. I was clear of the city traffic when Barry called back. He related that he found several areas where marble to golf ball size clumps of fertilizer were still present on the pasture. He even saw a cow walk up and eat one of the small clumps.

Barry explained that Mr. Earnest and he had been offered a price reduction on the fertilizer because it had gotten wet in storage and could not be used as customary in mechanical crop planters. Barry now realized that the moisture had made the fertilizer clump and, as a result, it would stop up the flow in the planters. The clumping likewise allowed the fertilizer to be more easily consumed by curious cows. It appeared we had found the answer to the death losses at his farm – he "fertilized the cows."

The next steps were to minimize any further losses and to prove that the fertilizer was the cause of death. I instructed Barry to move his herd to another pasture that had not received fertilizer. This would minimize any further exposure to nitrates. A rain or two would solubilize the fertilizer and wash it into the soil making the pasture safe again in the near future. I also called Mr. Earnest to tell him of the situation and get him to move his cows to a clean pasture. He was unaware of any death losses and thanked me for notifying him.

Nitrates cause death by starving the brain and body of oxygen. The nitrates are absorbed from the digestive system into the blood stream and convert hemoglobin in the red blood cells into methemoglobin. The methemoglobin does not carry and release oxygen to the tissues like normal hemoglobin. Nitrate poisoning may cause death within one-half hour to four hours after symptoms appear. Symptoms usually appear when methemoglobin reaches 30 to 40 percent, and death occurs when methemoglobin reaches 80 to 90 percent.

As Barry astutely observed, a symptom of nitrate toxicity is rapid, heavy breathing as the cow tries to compensate for the blood's inability to oxygenate the tissues. Nitrates are difficult to find in the blood after death because postmortem changes rapidly mask its presence. The one place that is not rapidly affected postmortem is the ocular fluid in the eye. Therefore, I instructed Barry to find a syringe and needle and withdraw ocular fluid from the eye of several of the dead cows. These ocular fluid samples were to be taken immediately to the state diagnostic laboratory for testing. This process would be the quickest and easiest way to prove that the fertilizer was the cause of death. I would use my cell phone to call ahead and set up the testing. Once the samples were submitted to the diagnostic lab nothing else needed to be done until I returned home and the lab reported the results.

The next morning the lab reported that the ocular fluid samples were positive for nitrates. I called Barry to inform him of the results and asked him to get me in touch with the fertilizer company that sold and spread the fertilizer. About an hour later the manager of the fertilizer company called my cell phone. We spoke for a few minutes and he agreed to take responsibility for the dead cows. They carried insurance for accidents like this. A good faith gesture such as this showed the farming community that the company cared about their businesses and would treat them fairly. In the future they would not spread clumped fertilizer on pastures occupied by cows to avoid "fertilizing the cows." As an aside note, I never saw any of the affected cows. This whole problem was resolved over the cell phone.

**

The story above makes it sound like nitrate problems in cattle are rare accidents. In actuality, this case of "fertilizing the cows" was not the way I typically encountered nitrate toxicity in cattle. I have seen many more cases of toxicity resulting from forages and water than from direct exposure to fertilizer.

Numerous forages in the cow's diet can accumulate nitrates in toxic amounts given the right conditions. These nitrate accumulators include popular pasture grasses like sorghums, sudangrass, pearl millet, as well as fescues if they are over-fertilized or experience abrupt stoppages of growth. Conditions such as drought, herbicide damage, late afternoon heat wilting, heavy fertilization with animal manures, and even periods of several cloudy days can contribute to nitrate buildup. These same stress conditions cause some common weeds like pigweed, pokeweed, and Johnsongrass to accumulate nitrates.

Nitrates persist in plant tissues when haying. I have been involved numerous times when high nitrate hays were purchased without testing beforehand. Usually, the hays originated from farms applying large quantities of liquid manures (hog farms). If one produces his own hay or is considering cutting a drought stressed crop for hay or silage, consider a nitrate test first, and especially if the crop received heavy fertilization.

Nitrates also can be found in water, because nitrates are very soluble in water. Nitrates move readily in surface water and this is one of the reasons why nitrogen needs to be applied every year to most forage crops—nitrates leach out! Where do you think the nitrates go? Many times it is into the groundwater.

I had a favorite dairy client family in central North Carolina with a persistent low level herd fertility problem. We tested for everything— eight different infectious diseases, five different mycotoxins, also feed toxins such as nitrates, poor semen quality, poor AI technique, and even the phases of the moon. We frustratingly came up with no answers. As a last resort we ran a water quality test and finally found the source of the fertility problem that we were pursuing.

The farm had a low level of nitrates in the well water. Low levels of nitrate exposure will not typically kill an adult cow, because the rumen micro-flora will metabolize it to safer compounds, and the cow can actually compensate by increasing her respiratory rate. But, fetuses are not ruminants yet, and with their rapid growth, they cannot survive the low oxygen levels that nitrates often generate. The low blood oxygen levels lead to early embryonic death which resembles infertility.

After putting a water treatment system on the well to remove the nitrates, the herd infertility problem disappeared. The farmer was again enabled to "fertilize the cows" at a normal conception rate. Importantly, the farmer and his family also used the same contaminated well as the dairy herd. As a side note, the farmer's daughter-in-law presented him with his first grandchild after the treatment system was fitted to the well. Hmm?

CHAPTER 32
An Anaplasma Solution Outlawed

I was on the roof of my family's little lake place, the "Galphin Getaway," tarring holes in the tin roof one summer morning when my cell phone rang. The caller was a panicking client, Mike, who had found two dead cows in his dairy housing area at Mapleview Dairy. He had two other cows down and unable to rise in the same area. He needed me to immediately come and determine the cause of illness. In order to help me reach a diagnosis, he had already called the diagnostic lab and loaded one of the dead cows for transport there. He would let me know what the state lab found. I explained where I was and what I was doing and apologized for not being able to arrive quickly. The "Galphin Getaway" was two hours from his farm.

I managed to slow him down enough to ask a few questions before he drove off to the lab, knowing he would be hard to question while he was at the lab. I asked him what the ages of the affected animals were. They were all adults in the milking string in early lactation but not recently postpartum (not recently calved). I asked him to look at the mucous membranes (eyes and lips) for paleness or discoloration and to take the temperature of the affected live cows. In his observations the cows were pale and yellowish with no elevated fever. None of the affected cows had any current or previous health problems since their calving. These observations made little sense to me at this time. I would need to more closely examine the herd and run some tests.

Just out of caution, I asked him to get the laboratory doctor to do a special procedure called a liver impression smear and look at it under a microscope. Quite often acute deaths to a blood disease called Anaplasmosis were missed on autopsies due to blood clotting changes that this test could circumvent. He wrote all this down and rushed off to transport the dead cow to the laboratory about 20 miles from his farm. I climbed down from my rooftop and changed from my lake shorts into my farm coveralls. I left the "Galphin Getaway" located in northeastern North Carolina for a diagnostic adventure in Orange County, North Carolina.

When I arrived at Mapleview Dairy one of the down cows had just died. I quickly examined it and drew a blood sample. Then I examined the other down cow finding pale yellow mucous membranes in both animals. I noted only slight elevation of body temperature in the cows and this could have been due to the increasing summer ambient temperature. Nothing else remarkable was found in any of the affected cows – only signs of anemia (low red blood cells) and icterus (yellowing due to destruction of red cells). My suspicions of the blood disease Anaplasmosis were greatly heightened by what I had seen on physical exams.

Not long after I finished the physical exams, Mike returned from the laboratory. He shared that the lab doctor would call me as soon as he had finished the autopsy and summarized his findings. Mike anxiously asked me if I had any ideas of what was going on and how he could minimize his losses.

I told Mike I suspected Anaplasmosis, a blood disease of cattle that was either spread by ticks or the direct transfer of blood from an infected cow to an uninfected cow. I asked if there was any way blood could have been transferred between cows because it was unusual for dairy cows to have many ticks in a modern facility. Mike's face turned red and he admitted that they had begun injecting all the fresh cows (recently calved) with the drug oxytocin during milking. Oxytocin helped milk letdown and increased milk yield.

The farm had just started doing this oxytocin treatment and had been using the same needle for all the cows until they could buy some new ones. I asked if the farm had purchased any new cows recently that might have been infected. He stated that they often participated in good cattle sales, so they might have bought a problem animal unaware. These admissions of a method of introduction and a method of spread made me even more suspicious of Anaplasmosis. Suddenly, the cell phone rang and it was the laboratory doctor with information that the liver impression smear revealed what he thought were Anaplasmosis organisms, called marginal bodies, in the red blood cells.

My diagnosis was verified.

Mike and I used the next hour to develop a treatment and management plan for the herd. I had done this for numerous herds over the past 45 years, but only rarely were dairy farms involved. We immediately stopped using shared needles for the oxytocin treatment. We also instructed everyone to be on alert for animals with signs of weakness or respiratory distress. Affected animals were to get immediate attention.

The disease can be treated using tetracycline antibiotics. The plan was to take a blood sample on all the adult cows. When blood test results were completed we would dry off any positive cows which were close to the end of lactation, and also treat them with injectable tetracyclines. Then we would feed tetracyclines to the dry cow herd in their ration to ensure no carrier animals would freshen or calve still carrying the disease.

For the remaining lactating cows, we would either sell or isolate and treat the positive ones, allowing us to discard their milk for an appropriate time. Lastly, we would retest the herd after the first winter frost, as soon as the tick vector season was over, to be sure we had identified all positive animals. We would then treat or remove any remaining animals identified as positive on these winter test results.

Mike was good with all these plans and ready to start the very next day. However, on the next morning when I arrived I found Mike's wife's favorite show cow to be gravely ill due to anemia and weakness. Without a blood transfusion she would die. I found suitable young bovine blood donors and collected eight quarts of blood. This blood was then infused intravenously into the show cow's jugular vein and as the treatment progressed, she improved in condition. The treatment of the valuable show cow ran late into the day, resulting in a delay of the herd blood testing. Consequently, the following day we bled the entire milking and dry cow herds, a total of about 160 cows. I filled in the laboratory submission paperwork overnight and submitted the blood samples the next morning.

There were 18 positive cows found in the herd. Mike sold four of them and dried off two. I showed Mike and his herdsman how I preferred to treat the cows and helped them with the first of four injections. The milk from these cows was discarded or withheld from the salable milk tank for 10 days because tetracycline antibiotics would be present in the milk. Before any treated cow's milk was kept for sale, the milk was tested negative for all antibiotics.

All of these procedures and the milk discard were very expensive, costing about $400 each for 14 infected cows. Add to this cost the death of three cows and the blood transfusion and you get a loss of over $11,000. No more animals died after the treatment began but, as you will soon understand, this was not the end of the trouble.

After the first frost, about three months later, we scheduled another herd blood test. I drew the blood samples in the morning and immediately took the blood to the lab only 20 minutes away. The laboratory set up the tests straight away while I finished the submission paperwork. The results were ready the next morning and held a surprise. There were 24 positives found. Eight of the positive cows were not a surprise because they had been treated earlier and expectedly retained an immune titer to the disease. The surprise was that 16 were supposedly new infections.

This was hard to believe since we had made every effort to stop the spread of the disease by using new needles and syringes on all injections and treating positive animals. And also, there had been no new clinical cases for over three months. Therefore, I questioned the lab's results and asked for a retest of the blood. I explained to the lab that I had seen false positive tests before in Mississippi when the samples were tested too soon after being drawn. The false positives resulted from an immune protein called complement that needed three hours "wait time" to be inactivated before tests were run. The laboratory personnel countered that this was a new, different test and the directions did not call for any "wait time." The lab refused to retest the samples as a matter of policy, but they did give me the telephone number of the Anaplasmosis test kit manufacturer.

I called the test kit maker that day to ask if they would rerun the tests. They found the request and justification of the rerun of the tests intriguing and consented to the rerun. So, I called the state lab and asked them to mail the blood samples to the manufacturer, and they did so. Meanwhile, Mike had to decide what to do with the positive test result cows, because Christmas holidays were approaching. He decided not to wait on the new test rerun and to isolate, treat, and discard milk from the positive cows while he had enough help to do the treatment. He did not understand the confusion over the test results and just wanted to be done with the problem before Christmas, even though it would be very expensive to discard all the milk from ten percent of his herd.

In about a week I had the newly rerun results which showed only two new cows were positive. I reported this to Mike and he was actually relieved that the problem had not been as bad as it appeared. I had been correct to doubt the earlier tests and to pursue answers to the high positive rates. The manufacturer contracted with us to do some more blood testing in Mike's herd in conjunction with the state laboratory and found that indeed the test required a "wait time" or incubation time before running the blood. They thanked us for bringing this to their attention and changed the test kit instructions to prevent further false positives. The manufacturer also promised to publish these findings in an appropriate journal, but to my knowledge there has been no public disclosure of the test problems published.

Mike and I discussed this herd Anaplasmosis problem at length and he thanked me for quickly diagnosing the disease and setting a management plan in motion. I apologized for the losses of milk that were unnecessary due to testing errors. There would be no way to recover those losses. Fortunately, the farm was in good financial condition and was able to withstand the blow. I felt gratified that we had resolved Mike's disease problem with minimal animal losses and that I had pursued the erroneous test results. These actions reduced the potential for future industry losses due to false positive test results.

In a look back, one of the keys to removing the disease from Mike's herd was the use of a mineral mix in the dry cow (non-lactating) ration. The short course of intravenous tetracycline treatment we used on lactating cows reduced a cow's clinical infection and infectivity for herd mates. But, it was not sufficient to remove the carrier state of the disease from every cow. Removing the carrier state required a much longer course of treatment which the ration mineral inclusion provided. We completely removed the disease from the herd by feeding the tetracycline mineral for over a year in the dry (non-lactating) herd.

I had created this mineral formulation 45 years earlier when I joined the faculty at Mississippi State as a consequence of being assigned the task of removing Anaplasmosis from the university herds. I used the tetracycline mineral for over four decades to safely treat animals for Anaplasmosis. The mineral was sometimes fed free choice and sometimes included in a mixed ration, but it had always been an effective tool against Anaplasmosis. I used it over and over to treat and eliminate the disease from cattle herds throughout the southeastern states.

Two years after the problem in Mike's herd the United States Food and Drug Administration (FDA) changed regulations and made it very difficult to continue using this mineral in a convenient way. Actually it is hard to find a mineral company that is even interested and willing to manufacture the mineral. I hope nobody tells Anaplasmosis about this development!.

CHAPTER 33
Vende Latte, LLC – School Milk Vending

I have previously written about the importance of industry advocacy in the story of the "*Belligerent Longhorn.*" An entrepreneurial dairy client whose wife taught high school came to me with an idea for a milk vending business in schools. This idea was bursting with industry advocacy in my assessment. There were a few hitches, however. He wanted me to set up the business structure, provide the funding, procure the vending machines, order the milk, and find the suitable school markets. He would own 50 percent of the business and do all the hands-on work of stocking the vending machines and collecting the money. I thought about it and realized that this project would allow us to introduce a healthy, wholesome food choice into the food vending areas of schools where only unhealthy choices currently existed. I agreed with his terms, since there should be minimal valuable time required from me. After all, what could go wrong with such a noble industry advocacy project, right?

So, I organized a business named Vende Latte, LLC, which means in Italian "it sells milk" to honor my Italian dairy connections. Next, I explored milk vending machines and surprisingly found them to be quite expensive, about $5000 each. I ordered five of these machines to start. Then, I began looking for a source of long shelf-life milk and settled on a company in Arizona with several good flavors of 90 day ultra-pasteurized milk.

Finally, I began contacting schools. I could never get in to speak with an official at a local Wake County public school; not even at the high school where my son attended. The local private schools were easier to connect with and welcomed the milk machines because many of them had no cafeterias and students brought their lunches. Soon the screw topped bottles of milk and the vending machines were delivered. I helped my dairyman partner put the machines in place and we were off and running with our little Vende Latte business. We placed machines in one public high school in a rural county and in four private schools in the Raleigh area.

After one month of business I began to answer the question of what could go wrong with this industry advocacy project. The rural school and the most expensive private school had machines in unsupervised areas and there were small groups of "thugs" in the schools that continually vandalized the machines for money or free milk. The school administrators would not let us secure the machines in any way, so the machines had to be removed and placed in two other private schools. Things were going well in the other private schools with the exception that my dairy partner was in the middle of corn harvest season and could not take time to properly service all the machines as promised. I stepped up to help since I was at risk for all the money invested in the business. I quickly began to look forward to the end of harvest season while I kept on filling milk machines.

To my astonishment, after several months in just 5 schools, the Wake County Public Health Department called me in for a meeting. The assistant director had heard about our work in the private schools and was impressed with our business model and results. She asked if we would be willing to place machines in the Wake County Public School System because no one else was trying to do this good work. I explained to her that we had tried, but had not had any success connecting with the Wake County Public Schools, even though my children attended. She explained that with her help I would be able to place the machines in the schools.

Her motivation was for health purposes. She quoted statistics showing an alarming increase in type two diabetes in school children. It was her belief that the schools should offer healthy food choices in the vending areas where presently there were no such choices. These were the only food areas open all day when cafeterias were closed. Health class teaches that students should make healthy snack choices and then we don't offer them.

I was impressed with her logic and sincerity and agreed to work with Wake County schools. The Wake County Public School System (WCPS) is the largest in the state of North Carolina and the third largest school system in the United States, so I immediately ordered more milk machines for greater industry advocacy.

Then the runarounds began. I was finally able to pinpoint the reason for WCPS's reluctance to cooperate. The school system finance officer let it slip that WCPS had a six million dollar contract with a soft drink bottling company. The finance officer warned me not to interfere, but I was determined to get to the root of the problem. I contacted the local bottler and got an appointment with the manager. He was very professional and explained that they had no product which milk would compete with, so he was "okay" with the milk vending machines. I asked him to write a letter to that effect, but he declined my request saying that he would do so if the school system requested it.

I thought I was making progress until I revisited the WPCS finance officer and asked him to write a letter to the bottler to request a letter that would allow him to write other letters to the school principals authorizing the placement of milk vending machines. The finance officer refused to write the letter stating that I had no authority to request such an action from him. I explained to him that I was asked by the county public health department to place the milk machines in WCPS schools and I represented them in this request. He refused and requested a letter from them.

I made an appointment with the Assistant Director of Wake County Public Health Department. At the meeting, I requested she write a letter to the WCPS finance officer requesting him to write a letter to the local bottler requesting a letter stating there was no conflict with the current contract so that the finance officer could write letters to school principals authorizing the placement of milk machines in vending areas. This was just as she, the assistant director, had originally requested of Vende Latte.

My heart sank when she refused to write the letter. I asked her if she still thought this was the right thing to do, and she acknowledged it was. But with only one year to retirement, she was afraid to get involved. This cowardly copout greatly angered me, so I stated that I had only one choice left, and that was to go to the court of public opinion. I was taking this to the local television investigative reporter through a friend I knew at the station. Maybe the television station could cut through the bureaucracy.

I was interviewed on television in front of a vending machine at one of the cooperating private schools. I gave my usual explanation of the need for healthy food choices in all schools, not just the private schools. However, the public schools would not authorize the milk machines. The investigative reporter then interviewed the WCPS finance officer, and he allowed that the public school system would now authorize the milk machines. After he stated this on the public airwaves, I thought the battles were finally over. But he called all the school principals and told them to ignore my visits and requests. I was never allowed to speak to any of the principals after numerous visits to schools.

Most people would have stopped trying much earlier than this, so, I would not have been blamed for giving up at this point. I did not give up. I couldn't understand why the principals were so willing to snub me to the point of not even meeting with me. So, I got another friend who was a friend of a principal to invite him to lunch and query him. My friend was to ask why principals were so attached to the bottler. What he found was that the school's portion of the soft-drink vending revenues was considered "undesignated funds." This meant the principals could spend it on anything they wished for, even if they shouldn't. Well, that explained a lot. The principals and the school system were just protecting their own slush funds and were willing to sacrifice student health for money.

With this information and the realization that my partner was never going to restart servicing the machines as promised, I made the decision to just get out of Vende Latte, LLC. I fortunately sold the machines and equipment for what was owed and shut it down. But, I still believed healthy choices in the schools was the right thing to do.

A few months later, I discovered a federal law called the "Child Nutrition and Integrity Act." It was passed unanimously by both the House of Representatives and the Senate and signed by President George Bush (tell me when this has happened since). The bill was written after a soft-drink bottling company sued an Arizona school for putting milk vending machines in schools. Our elected officials were so incensed by this attack on child health that they gave the state Department of Agriculture the authority to hold up school lunch funds if schools did not have healthy choices in vending areas with soft drinks. School lunch funds are a much larger pot of money than the soft drink contracts! I took this new but little-known law to the newly elected North Carolina Agriculture Commissioner and got his agreement to enforce its provisions.

The schools now have healthy choices in the vending areas, but the schools had to buy the machines and stock them because there was no one willing to trust that they would adhere to the law. I had lost all the battles in this war over healthy choices but the war had been won. I am optimistic that the children are the real winners.

CHAPTER 34
More Industry Advocacy

One of the most difficult times in my life came in January 2003. I have explained that my passion in life is feeding people and I worked mostly with dairymen to increase their efficiency in producing milk. In 2003 the financial pressures of the dairy market were very punishing. On a herd visit to a friend and client of 22-plus years I experienced a severe shock as my friend committed suicide while I was at his farm.

His wife told me later that he waited for me to arrive because he knew I would take care of his family in his absence. He had reached the end of his means to survive in the milk industry, or so he thought. His last resort to save his father-in-law's farm and provide for his family's future was through life insurance. The insurance did pay, because he had the courage to wait long enough to be vested in the insurance before he pulled the trigger.

I cannot fathom the mental and physical anxiety he must have endured as he secretly contemplated and carried out his plan. I deeply regret that our friendship was not close enough for him to have shared some of his problems before he finished his scheme. As his friend, I held his weeping wife until I could get most of her family together and gathered around her. And then, I drove 200 miles to pick up their son from college so that he would not try to drive home to his family farm with this untimely death on his mind. I brought him home to grieve with his mother, his two sisters, his grandparents, other family members, and also me.

This friend was a good dairyman but he had no control over his prices. You see, regardless of how efficient production is, the greatest determinant of profitability is the price you get paid for your product. The price he was receiving was set by the milk handlers in the industry.

The handlers, milk processors and milk coops, work very hard and smart to limit their competition so they can be more profitable. A group of milk handlers had gotten together (colluded) and eliminated most of the competition in milk sales and most of the competition for the purchase of raw milk. Free markets require competition to insure a fair and sustainable price and the colluding handlers were suppressing raw milk prices by eliminating competition. I will call this group of colluding handlers the "Cartel." This market activity is actually unlawful because it results in a monopoly of a marketplace. The adage "capitalism without competition is exploitation" was very true in the dairy market. Dairymen and their families were being exploited. I was so profoundly provoked by this whole situation that I determined to try and stop further exploitation of dairy families.

I began by convincing some lawyers and influential dairy producers that there was a need for this "Cartel" to be challenged in a class action suit over violation of antitrust laws. Litigations are not for the faint of heart. People and businesses get injured in lawsuits emotionally, reputationally, and financially whether one wins or loses. I have never sued anyone, and even in this instance, was unable to participate because I was not a dairy owner at the time. Nonetheless, I was certain that this was the only way to stop the exploitation of milk producers.

Antitrust laws were used to break up the big oil, steel, and railroad monopolies in the 1900s. A single individual would find it difficult to legally challenge a cartel, but a class action suit is a litigation filed on behalf of a group of injured plaintiffs. The suit was referred to as the Southeast Dairy Litigation.

A class action suit has multiple types of plaintiffs and defendants. The named plaintiffs were individual dairymen, half of which were my clients. The injured class was the total of the Southeastern dairymen. The individually named defendants were "Cartel" organization's officers; and the injuring defendants were the businesses of the "Cartel."

Actually, the United States Justice Department (DOJ) had begun to look into the "Cartel's" antitrade activities years earlier but the investigation was stopped by the U. S. Attorney General, who had some connections to the "Cartel" officers. Even after we obtained this (DOJ) investigation's information through the Freedom of Information Act as a jumpstart, it still took almost 10 years to get the case into the courtroom.

The good thing about the long pretrial period is that I had the opportunity to enter the dairy business again and become a member of the plaintiff-injured class. This allowed me to participate directly in the suit and testify in the class action fairness hearing. These following excerpts are taken from my testimony in the fairness hearing.

> *Your Honor, the manipulation of milk supplies and prices carried out by these defendants does more than just affect the prices at stores. It affects the livelihood of many dairymen and rural communities. The North Carolina Department of Agriculture calculated that $14 million were removed from the NC dairy market in just one year, and this case covers ten years for twelve southeastern states. One defendant CEO named in this suit received, in addition to his salary, over $110 million, another CEO got $130 million, and another took $80 million just for themselves individually. The money that these defendant conspirators and co-conspirators extracted from the market for themselves—by my count (as recorded in this litigation) is over $1.5 billion.*

I spoke further,

> *The greed of these defendants and the games they played with milk prices financially stressed the producers in the Southeast. I personally hold the defendants in this suit complicit in the death of my friend and in the ruining of many other dairymen who have exited the industry in the last 15 years. Dairy numbers have declined from 1,200 in North Carolina in the 1980s when I moved to the area to less than 200 today. In South Carolina, another state I work in, the numbers have gone from 800 to less than 100. And the damage doesn't stop at the dairies. The milk truck drivers lose their jobs, tractor dealers lose, local feed dealers close, the rural electric loses, the local bank loses, all laborers on the farm lose their jobs, the veterinarian loses, and the local church loses. What these defendants did to rural America is not moral.*

At this point, I proceeded to explain my objections to the settlement offers:

> *There is ample evidence presented in this case to show that the*

changes which were made in the market created terrible problems for the dairymen in the Southeast. I am not going into the specifics of those actions at this point. There is also ample evidence shown in the case arguments to justify the need for additional court mandated market changes to provide relief and protection for the Southeast dairymen. Without such market changes the industry will not survive. It is the lack of market changes in this settlement that I object to, not the amount of the monetary settlement that the lawyers have carved out for themselves. I offer the following points to be included in the settlement.

At this juncture, I offered a list of 10 market changes that would go a long way toward healing the Southeastern milk market. I will not describe them in this book because of the lengthy explanations required for readers to understand them; however, I will move on to highlight more important parts of the testimony.

Your Honor, this settlement makes the lawyers happy, but it does not go far enough, at least not far enough to secure the future of the Southeastern dairy industry. The requested market changes must be a part of this settlement or the case should go to trial. I know I am the lone objector to the current settlement discussion, and remarkably, I am the originator of the suit. I ask that a committee be formed to study these requested market changes and try to find a way to get them into the final settlement. If necessary I'll find out how to file a Notice of Appeal if the settlement continues to exclude market changes because for 10 years I've carried the burden of my friend's untimely and unnecessary death.

The judge then asked the following question:

I understand all of the things you asked for, all the points you've made. This case has been divided into two litigations, and a large dairy cooperative is not a part of the first settlement. Realistically speaking, without that coop defendant at the table, can all of those things you asked for be accomplished? This first settlement involves a monetary payment by only two of the defendants. Can all those things you're asking for be accomplished through this settlement with only these defendants?

I responded as follows:

> *Your Honor, the current settlement as written does not divest them (the "Cartel") of any of their processing plants. They still control the milk market in the Southeast. They still have control of 51 out of 54 milk processing plants in the Southeast, if I'm not mistaken. I don't see the market changing because some corporation paid a $150 million settlement. I didn't go into the specific actions of individually named defendants as detailed in the court record, but at least one individually named person, in this case, has taken as much as $180 million out of the cooperatives in just one insider joint venture. So, this settlement, based on my calculations, is a drop in the bucket when compared to the $1.2 billion skimmed away from the dairymen over the past 10 years.*

> *So, in answer to your question, I don't think the settlement goes far enough to keep this group of defendants from destroying the Southeastern dairy industry. I'm not pleading for my own sake. This is not about me. This is about the friends and families I've had the privilege to know and serve over a 35-year veterinary career. I watched them endure the market abuse, and all along, I hoped that the future would be different so that this industry could do its part in feeding the world's exploding population because my passion is feeding the world. If these defendants continue running the dairymen out of business, we will not be able to do the required doubling of the food supply that will be necessary in the next 30 years.*

> *I don't want my children and grandchildren to live in a world where enough food is not available for all people. I pray they won't live in a world like that. Without the requested market changes my expectation is that within five years the "Cartel", the defendants, will succeed in taking all the money in this settlement back out of the dairymen's paychecks. Your Honor, you have seen the evidence in the record and you understand that the Defendants know how to get the money back. The settlement needs to go further than just money to make the market competitive again.*

The Judge responded, "All right. I understand your position. Thank you very much. You may retake your seat."

After this exchange I left the court and returned to my dairy and veterinary businesses in North Carolina. In the following days the effects of my testimony became evident. There was a call from a journalist friend informing me that she had written a piece in a national journal complimenting my stand and stating that "in a normally noisy, bustling courtroom one could hear a pin drop as the testimony implicated the defendants in the death of a friend and client." Next came a taped interview with NPR (National Public Radio) that was broadcast all over the nation. Friends from the Midwest and West Coast called saying they had heard the broadcast. The New York Times even did a telephone interview that was used in a first page article. The message was out and the pressure was on. My advocacy was successful!

The Judge approved the first settlement as written; however, he made sure that many of the requested market changes were included as part of the second settlement. The total settlement cost the "Cartel" $300 million. Plaintiff lawyers were paid one–third of the total. Today, three of the "Cartel" businesses no longer exist, and the remaining "Cartel" members are in litigation against each other. The Southeast Dairy Litigation severely weakened the "Cartel." Almost immediately, dairymen in the Northeast filed the Northeast Dairy Litigation which was eventually successful also. There are still some problems in the dairy markets, but there is no longer a powerful "Cartel" orchestrating all of the exploitation.

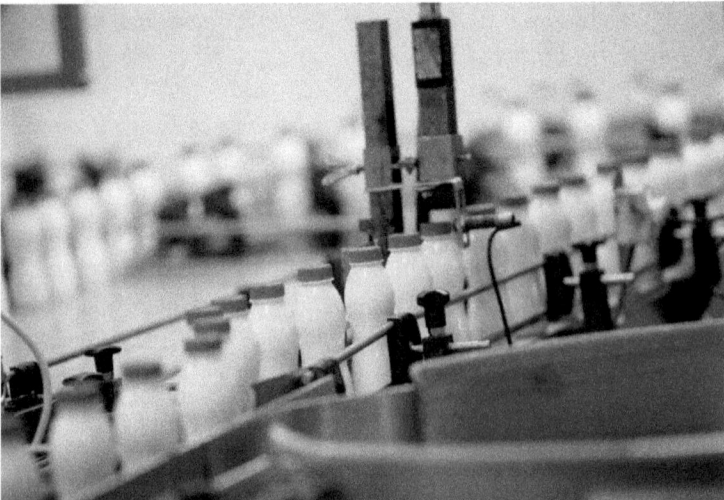

It is indeed unfortunate that none of the crooked individually named defendants ever paid any price for the damage they did to others while stealing from the industry. These smart crooks induced the compromised corporate boards of directors to indemnify (compensate) them for all of their court costs and penalties. As predicted, dairymen from the large coop were eventually on the hook for a substantial part of the second settlement, but the market changes helped them pay for it.

CHAPTER 35
The Tail Swiper

Oh my, she was a real beauty! Tall with perfect legs and her face was angelic. Her long eyelashes curled slightly upward and her eyes were large and bright. Her rump was broad and her tail had a large white switch on the end that hung at the level of her hocks. She was the best pedigreed heifer we had ever bred. She had so much potential. I had anticipated doing embryo transfers from her to start a superior bloodline in our herd.

However, when she calved there was no milk. All four of her teats were closed tightly with no visible opening. The udder was painfully tight but no milk could be removed. I anesthetized her and tried to find an opening in the teats, but the teat ends and the entire two inch long steak canals were scarred shut. We had to sell her at the market. What a disappointment!

I was determined to find out what caused the teat scarring in my favorite heifer. My plan was to observe and photograph heifer's teat ends at many of my client's dairies and to interview my clients about similar problems in their cattle. I found out that many of them had heifers calving with one or more blind teats every year, usually in the summer time of the year. I reviewed the literature to find reports of the problem in other regions and found that the further south a farm was located, the greater the incidence of the problem.

I also began to realize from the literature that the problem of heifer teat scarring had some similarity to "summer mastitis" in dry dairy cows, a disease which was being reported in British veterinary journals. The shared causation in heifer teat damage and "summer mastitis" was the presence of the similar common bacterial infections. These bacteria are usually found in the cattle environment or on their skin, but it is unusual to have the bacteria inside the teat or udder of non-milking animals.

My search for the method of introduction of bacteria into the non-lactating udder led me to realize that common biting flies were the fomites (carriers of infection) in the heifer and dry cow infections. The seasonal relationship of highest infection incidence correlated well with the period of greatest numbers of biting flies. I was able to photograph biting flies on the teats of heifers during the summer months at all of my client herds. In many cases the small teats were crusted over with blood and scabs from the numerous fly bites.

The head and shoulders are the typical sites of preference for most biting pests of cattle. However, the use of fly repellant ear tags and sprays have moved the flies down to the animal's underbelly and the tender, unhaired teats. Flies can carry bacteria in their gut and deposit them on teats when they lacerate the teat during a blood meal. It did appear that the teat ends needed to be injured by the flies' feeding in order for the bacteria to fully colonize the teat prior to invading the teat sphincter. Since it is impossible to remove bacteria from the cattle environment, it became apparent that control of this costly disease complex would have to revolve around control of the fly vector on the udder. Control of the flies would require creating a special device.

I began crafting a unique pyrethroid insecticide dispensing device which could be fastened or glued to the tail of a heifer during the fly vector season. I called this device the "Tail Swiper." I made enough of the "Tail Swipers" to begin a "heifer mastitis complex" control experiment; and simultaneously I applied for a patent on the device. "Tail Swiper" tail tags were easy to apply and could be placed on the animals without even individually catching their heads in a chute. One could just line the heifers up in a narrow lane, reach over the top for their tail, apply glue, and apply the "Swiper."

When the initial study was completed the results were amazing. The "Tail Swiper" significantly ($P < .0001$ for those who care) reduced "heifer mastitis complex" in the treated group versus the control group with no swipers. I began sharing the initial study's new information with the veterinary and dairy industries. I published the study results in the Bovine Practitioner Journal and I lectured at various professional meetings. There was much excitement in the industry relating to the device. The patent was soon granted, and I began to get inquiries from a myriad of academicians and even a major animal health company.

Things were looking up for the MOO VET.

US005280768A

United States Patent [19]

Galphin, Jr.

[11] Patent Number: 5,280,768

[45] Date of Patent: Jan. 25, 1994

[54] METHOD OF PREVENTING MASTITIS USING INSECTICIDE DISPENSER ATTACHED TO COW'S TAIL

[76] Inventor: Samuel P. Galphin, Jr., 6509 Saddle Path Cir., Raleigh, N.C. 27606

[21] Appl. No.: 71,974

[22] Filed: Jun. 7, 1993

[51] Int. Cl.⁵ A01K 13/00
[52] U.S. Cl. 119/156
[58] Field of Search 119/156, 157, 159, 14.01, 119/14.02; 43/124, 131, 132.1

[56] **References Cited**

U.S. PATENT DOCUMENTS

2.688.311	9/1954	Pierce .	
4.430.961	2/1984	Steckel	119/156
4.562.794	1/1986	Speckman .	
4.574.742	3/1986	Morgan, Jr.	119/156
4.706.610	11/1987	Morgan. Jr. .	
4.878.456	11/1989	Howe	119/156
5.044.114	9/1991	Haberer	119/156

OTHER PUBLICATIONS

Nickerson et al. "Mastitis Control in Replacement Heifers", *Bovine Proceedings*, Jan. 1992. pp. 76–78.
Fox et al., "Heifer Mastitis", *National Mastitis Council Meeting Proceedings*, 1993 pp. 187–193.
Hoard's Dairyman, Aug. 1992. p. 3.
Heatmount Detector literature.
"Terminator" Ear Tag Container.

Primary Examiner—Gene Mancene
Assistant Examiner—Todd E. Manahan
Attorney, Agent, or Firm—John G. Mills

[57] **ABSTRACT**

This invention is a method of reducing the incidence of bovine mastitis by mounting an extended release insecticide dispenser on the ventral surface of the bovine's tail just cranial to the switch. This allows the insecticide vapors to permeate the area between the rear legs and the udder and its associated teats. This greatly reduces the incidence of biting insects which transmit mastitis causing bacteria to the teats. Also, tabs are provided on the extended release insecticide dispenser to hold the same in place on the tail until the adhering medium is cured. These tabs are preferably made from a moisture degenerative type material such as paper.

8 Claims, 2 Drawing Sheets

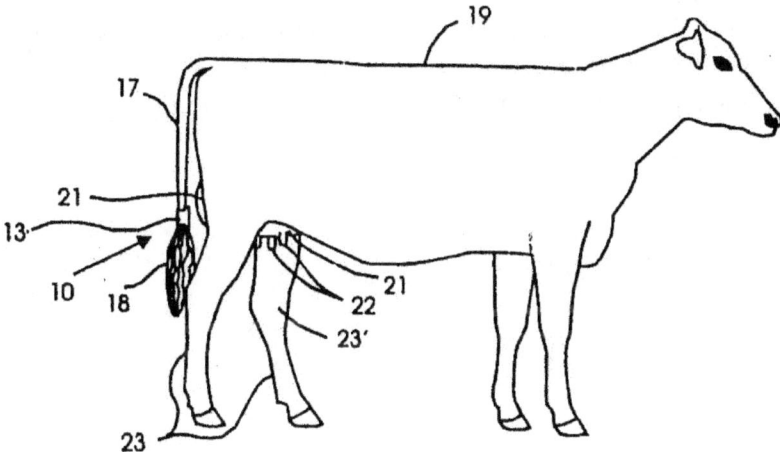

Copy of Tail Swiper Patent. Read more about this patent at
https://patents.justia.com/patent/5280768

In due course, I traveled to the headquarters of the major animal health company. We made a cooperation agreement for the company to manufacture the "Tail Swiper" and for me to continue to study and document the effectiveness of the swipers in preventing heifer mastitis. The "Tail Swipers" they made were superior to the ones I had made in my garage. With the new tail tags I was able to get studies going at several major universities headed up by well-known scientists.

One major southern university, LSU, found that the tags were even effective on beef cows and actually eliminated all the flies on the cattle as a result of the cows switching their "Swiper" loaded tails over their backs and sides. Things were really moving in a positive way until the results of that LSU study were published. The LSU study revealed that the "Tail Swiper" actually eliminated the need for other fly repellent devices such as ear tags. The major animal health company withdrew from our cooperation agreement and no other insecticide tag makers would work with the "Swiper" any longer, fearing that the "Swiper" would take away their market for cattle insecticide ear tags.

I was sorely disappointed in the animal health industry which would abandon such an effective device for preventing the costly heifer mastitis and summer mastitis in non-lactating cows out of fear for their market share. Their refusal to manufacture the "Swiper" left me with the undertaking of establishing an OSHA (Occupational Safety and Health Administration) and FDA (Food and Drug Administration) approved insecticide handling and manufacturing facility. At that time, the cost to do this was almost half of a million dollars. Sadly, I just had to allow the patent to expire for lack of time and funds. Too bad for the cattle and too bad for the MOO VET!

CHAPTER 36
Mechanical Mastitis at Caserta, Italy

As we motored over the mountain top in Caserta, Italy, I was impressed by the size and the complexity of the dairy farm located in the valley below. Worldwide Agriculture Consulting (WAC), the business Dr. Livio and I had founded, had just established a contract with Cirio, Polenghi, De Rica (CPD) to evaluate the farm they owned near Caserta, a small city near Naples. This was my first of dozens of visits to La Fagianeria, our new client's farm. I was given a tour of the entire grounds and soon realized that many of the buildings I had seen from the mountaintop were not related to dairy production, but were associated with milk processing, milk laboratory quality control, and milk bottling. The farm milked, housed, and fed over 1200 adult dairy cows. However, the complex also processed milk from hundreds of smaller farms in the region. As for the dairy animals owned by CPD at La Fagianeria, all these cows calved here and resided here, but the babies were transported to another farm to be reared to adulthood before returning here to calve. La Fagianeria was one of the largest dairy farms in Italy, and I was impressed!

As per my usual methods, I made notes about everything and asked many questions as I followed along on the tour. Dr. Livio struggled to keep up with all the translations. In the future, he would be able to leave me at the farm alone as I learned the language better and understood the culture, but presently he was careful to stay by my side. As I observed the facilities, the cattle, and the work being done, I noticed many areas that needed attention and held potential for increasing profits at the farm. My confidence that we could make a positive economic difference at this farm was building.

I gathered pages of notes and spent three days there writing a summary of all my findings. The ration was very complicated, so I doubted that the feeding was done properly. Feed samples were taken to get a better handle on this and a return visit would be needed to address the ration. Reproductive records indicated too many days in milk passed before the cows were pregnant. The breeding delay resulted in lower than desired milk production, but I preferred to deal with this later since this initial visit was in June when it would be difficult to improve reproduction during the heat of summer. Last but not least, the all-important milk somatic cell count (SCC), the measure of mastitis (udder infection) in the cows, was too high. I decided to focus on this udder health problem first since its metric, SCC, is the most easily monitored and I desired to make a quick improvement in some metric as a result of this visit.

My usual methodology was to write a report of my findings after any farm visit, so in the report I put off dealing with the feeding program pending sample analyses, and I put off dealing with the reproductive program until cooler temperatures would aid my progress. I therefore, emphasized the udder health program. Having observed very poor milking technique during my farm tour, I began by instructing the farm manager, Cesare, and the herdsmen in an improved milking technique. Back in America I had several copies of a videotape of the preferred milking technique produced for me in the Italian language. I used this videotape and a written Italian handout to do the training of the managers and I left a copy of both of these instructional aids with them for their use in training the milkmen.

The somatic cell count at the dairy was so high that the farm had installed centrifuges to spin some of the cells out of the milk, so that the milk would pass the health tests. I recommended that the centrifuges be shut down to get a true cell count and to remain off as much as possible because the centrifuges not only removed somatic cells, but also removed two liters of milk per cow daily from the milk harvest. Lastly, I recommended that the milking equipment be serviced more frequently. I cautioned that there was a component on their milking system called a pulsator that operated using a thin rubber diaphragm which needed regular servicing.

In the United States I had owned and run a dairy equipment dealership for the purpose of renovating inferior milking systems that were contributing to mastitis in my clients' herds. Mastitis or infections of the cow's mammary gland is the most costly disease in the dairy industry. Even today, worldwide losses of over $30 billion annually are attributed to this disease complex. The mastitis complex arises as a result of three potential contributing causes—the milkman, the environment, and the milking machine. Readers should recall and review the references to mastitis in other chapters (*No Holes Bored*).

One cannot adequately control mastitis levels without being able to evaluate milking machine function. I had tested hundreds of milking systems over a two decade period and had become familiar with numerous makes of dairy equipment. I knew the strengths and weaknesses of the machinery from many manufacturers. In La Fagianeria I had identified a type of vacuum pulsator that frequently caused problems for my dairymen in America when service intervals were too long. I explained that this vacuum pulsator had a thin rubber diaphragm inside which would fail if not replaced regularly, and that without properly functioning pulsation, mastitis would result. I had calculated the diaphragm needed changing in La Fagianeria every 30 to 45 days instead of their usual four to six month interval.

This was early along in my time consulting in Italy and my Italian language skills were very poor. Dr. Livio was required for onsite interpretation and he had his nephew Dr. Gabrielle translate the written reports I created. When we departed the farm I felt I had done my best to get WAC and CPD off to a good consulting relationship. I'd be sure of it, if there were some questions sent back to America after they received my translated written report. However, there were never any questions. I didn't know if we had done an excellent job or if they were content to ignore the recommendations that we gave.

In August I had my answer to this question – they had ignored the written recommendations. CPD contacted Dr. Livio in a panic over a severe herd mastitis outbreak. La Fagianeria was experiencing over fifteen (15) new mastitis cases each day and had been doing so for ten days. As much as 20 percent of the milk was being discarded and nothing they did seemed to help the bad situation! When questioned, it was admitted that they had not serviced the vacuum pulsators in the milking system as recommended, and it appeared that the pulsators were failing.

This is when I received my first lesson in Italian culture. The farm manager, Cesare, had not arranged for milking system service before the month of August. In Italy apparently the whole country goes on a vacation called "holiday" for one to two months starting the first of August. Now, not only the local milking machine service company was closed for holiday, but all of the service companies in the entire country were closed for holiday. Cesare could not get anyone to come service the milking equipment.

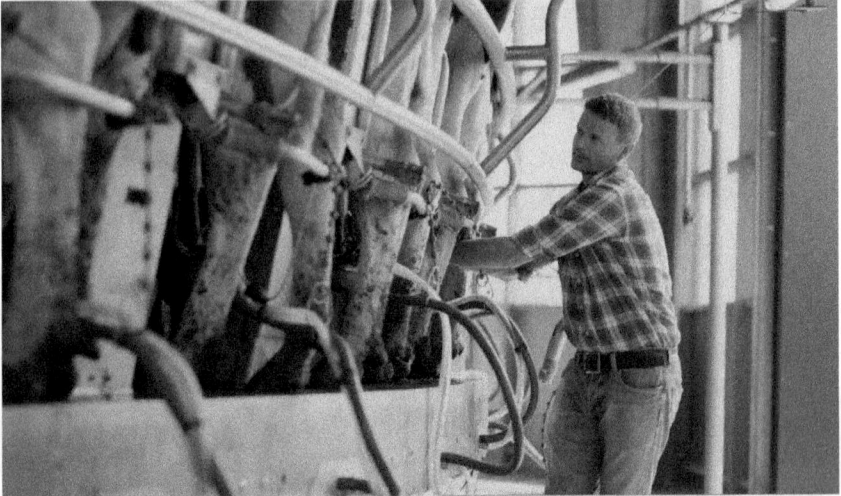

Milking Parlor in Operation

I also tried through international telephone calls to encourage a company to open up and help the farm, but this was futile. People in Italy take their holiday seriously. I finally resorted to calling the milking machine manufacturer's headquarters located in Sweden. The company headquarters arranged for a French team to travel to Caserta, Italy and do the required service on the failing milking equipment. After the repairs and service were completed, new mastitis cases immediately began to decrease. Cesare sent me a thank you note!

Unfortunately for Cesare, CPD administrators blamed him for the mastitis outbreak. He was fired from his management position. A new manager was hired and the new manager and I became fast friends over the next several years as we worked together to increase La Fagianeria's profitability. Cesare was hired by another large dairy farm that eventually contracted with Worldwide Agriculture Consulting to improve their farm's profitability. Fortunately, Cesare held no ill will towards me and we in time also became friends. One of the fond memories of my Italian consulting years was the memory of watching the Italian National Team win the World Cup Soccer Championship on Cesare's apartment television. He had prepared and served an authentic homemade Italian dinner for a small group of friends and invited me to participate in the festivities. From the balcony of his apartment we watched the people of Caserta victoriously dance in the streets below.

CHAPTER 37
Abortus in Buffalo–Italian Style

Brucellosis is a zoonotic disease which means it is passed from animals to humans. The organism that causes cattle brucellosis is named Brucella abortus after the Scottish microbiologist, Sir David Bruce. When cattle get brucellosis they get a little sick and if pregnant, they usually abort, and then they expose everyone, both cattle and humans, to highly infectious body fluids and excretions, including the milk. Brucella abortus is an intracellular bacteria making it nearly impossible to treat.

In humans the disease is called undulant fever for its characteristic recurring fevers. The majority of human cases have been associated with drinking unpasteurized milk or eating unpasteurized cheese, but there is also an occupational risk for those who work with cattle like milkmen, slaughter workers, and veterinarians. In the modern dairy industry pasteurization has made human cases rare and there are effective vaccines now to protect cattle.

Nonetheless, there are still pockets of the disease around the world, so commercial milk is tested negative by the Brucella milk ring test and young cows can be vaccinated to prevent infection. However, if a country has tested sufficiently and found no brucellosis, they can declare themselves free of Brucella and stop vaccinating. When I was working in Italy, Italy had declared itself free of brucellosis and no longer vaccinated. In contrast, America was still using vaccines.

You probably know where I'm going with all this discussion. I found brucellosis on one of the dairy cow farms I was consulting with in Italy. And, I suspected it in some of the other cow herds in Italy. What made me suspicious of brucellosis being present in this supposedly Brucella-free country was the high number of people reported in the daily newspaper who were found positive for Brucella by the public health department. The health department would weekly publish the names of Brucella infected people. (Can you imagine with our privacy laws in the US what would happen if the health department published people's names?)

The Italian public health officials usually attributed the infections to eating unpasteurized water buffalo cheese which is the authentic, traditional Italian mozzarella cheese. Yes, you heard me, real mozzarella cheese is made with water buffalo milk (mozzarella di Bufali) and is not pasteurized. The problem is that when water buffalo contract brucellosis they do not get sick or abort. They become inapparent carriers. As inapparent carriers the buffalo can have normal calves but have infected milk and infected birthing discharges. Many of these buffalo herds are housed and managed in the same regions that have cow dairies and can be sources of infection for cow herds by way of feral dogs and delivery vehicles.

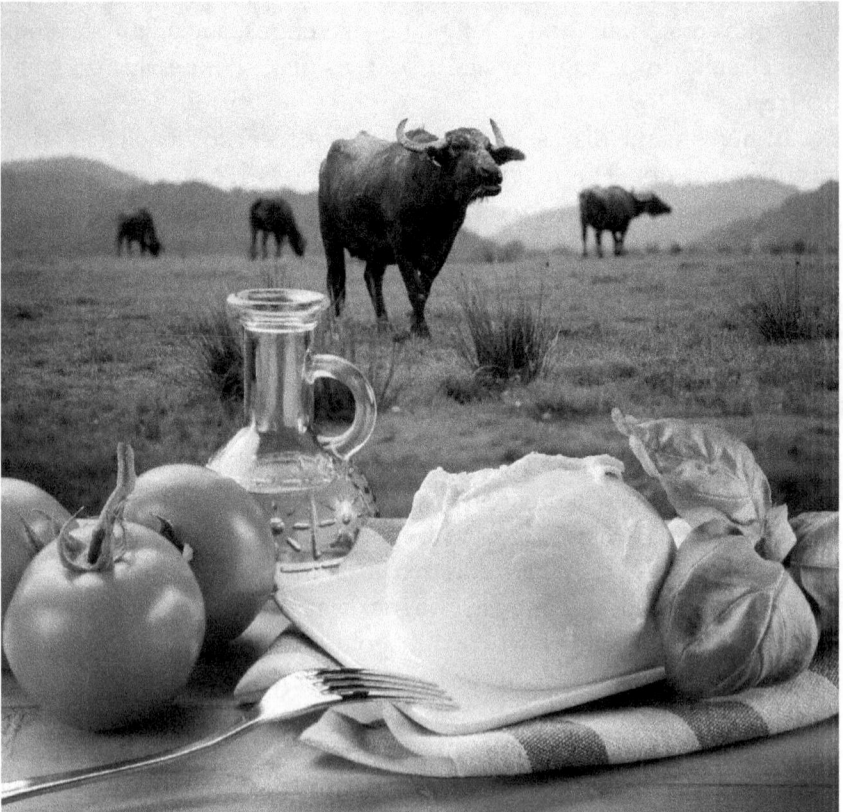

Mozzarella di Bufali

Together we looked at the herd records and observed an unusual number of recent abortions and stillbirths. It appeared that the abortions started in a remotely situated replacement heifer rearing facility located in a different region near numerous buffalo dairies. The pregnant heifers when they aborted were moved to the main farm to be milked. I was sure we had transported brucellosis to the milking herd also. I wasn't familiar with the law in Italy, but the law in America would have had the entire herd quarantined for testing and removal of positives. In America there would be strict sanitation measures instituted and restrictions would be placed on the sale of removed animals. It was time to have a serious meeting with the owners!

The owners of the farm were also processors of commercial milk. They wished to quietly handle the problem so that potentially bad press would not disrupt their market. They knew people who would help them with private testing and management of the disease. I realized I could do little to help with this problem, since I was only a consultant and not licensed to practice in Italy. I created a set of sanitation protocols for the herd and left the testing and removal of positives to the preference of owners.

I must admit that I continued to anxiously monitor the situation. I was scheduled to return to the farm in three months, so I began to research the possibility of using a newly developed vaccine that was being tested in America. Not surprisingly, I was contacted in just six weeks by the owners of the farm requesting an immediate return visit. Things had not been going well with their disease management program.

On arrival in Italy I was picked up at the airport and taken directly to the farm. Record review revealed an ongoing problem. At this time there were 40 positive cows being held in a quarantine pen waiting to go to slaughter. I asked why they did not send them directly to slaughter and the answer was that the beautiful fresh positive cows had been sent directly to slaughter initially, until it was discovered that some were being diverted for resale to local dairies. That's why they were now only selling cows that were completely dry (had no milk flow).

For me the resultant problem was that infected cows were kept on the farm for weeks with the risk of exposing others. They had already identified over 200 positive cows and sold them for about $500 each, when they were valued at $2,500. Losses from the disease were getting astronomical with the loss of milk, loss of cows, loss of calves, feeding positive cows, and also paying for the secret testing. In just a few months the cost had exceeded half a million dollars.

The testing was being done by Italian federal personnel from the Naples region, who were being paid in cash under the table. This was definitely illegal in the United States. In addition, five farm workers had been found to be infected with brucellosis by the local health department doctors who had assumed that the workers consumed unpasteurized buffalo cheese, since Italy was considered cow brucellosis free. This messy situation was so explosive that it was just about to blow up! The owners begged for me to find a safer, more effective solution.

Actually, I had been expecting to get more involved in controlling this Italian problem, so back in America I had been busy researching the new "RB-51" vaccine which had recently been put into use in America. The old vaccine called Strain-19 had some problems with safety for people, and problems with long term blood titers (positive tests) in vaccinated cows. I could not use a vaccine like the old one because it was not allowed in Italy and was not safe for people.

I knew the scientist that developed the new RB-51 vaccine and also had a veterinary friend in the USDA (United States Department of Agriculture) who was in charge of premarket test trials on the new vaccine. With their help I confirmed that this vaccine was very safe for people and animals, even if the cows were pregnant. And, the vaccine did not produce a blood titer that was detectable by currently used tests.

Also, importantly, the "RB-51" vaccine had been very effective in preventing disease in the American trials. The vaccine appeared to be perfect for this Italian situation, and I recommended immediate use to hopefully reverse the direction of the problems. However, there were a couple of problems to work out. The vaccine was only available in small five-dose containers, and Italy did not allow this vaccine nor vaccination for Brucellosis. The owners said to pursue this solution.

The next morning from Italy I telephoned my friend who developed the vaccine and asked him when the 25 dose vials would be ready. He reported that the USDA had just approved them and they would be made that week. I implored him to send the first five thousand doses to my office in North Carolina, and I would get them next week when I returned. The first problem was solved.

The second problem was more difficult. The owners said that I was allowed to ship the vaccine to the country of Paraguay where they had friends. They would be responsible after that and make arrangements to get the vaccine to Italy. This seemed to resolve the second problem, but I was skeptical about the transport program.

I gave them specific written recommendations for the use of the vaccine in heifers and in the milking cows. We would give all heifers one full dose immediately for full protection, but in the cows we would use one-fourth of a dose every three months for a year to ensure that no detectable blood titer was ever induced. It would be important to delay any official federal whole herd testing of the milking herd as long as possible, and we would continue to secretly blood test and remove positive cows and heifers. Lastly, I rewrote specific sanitation procedures and emphasized their implementation to protect humans from exposure until the incidence of the disease was nil. At the end of all these deliberations, I promised to return to Italy in four months if I was not wanted by the authorities.

In America, I found the vaccine had arrived at my office safely. I prepared the bottles for reshipping by removing the boxes and labels. I had left instructions for its use and didn't want any confusion. I telephoned the people in Paraguay to let them know when the package should arrive. I then waited for a call from Italy to let me know that the vaccine made it there and the program was underway.

This shipping process seemed a little surreptitious to my office manager (wife). She asked me if I was sure I was comfortable with possibly risking my license and our livelihood to please this client. After a little thought, I told her that I was doing this for the unsuspecting farm workers who were at risk and for the innocent cows facing slaughter. At this point there had been almost 600 valuable cows sent to slaughter! She accepted that I may have done a wrong thing for the right reason. I received the anticipated call from Italy that the vaccination program was underway so I kept my telephone lines open for any news until I revisited in three months.

On my return visit to Italy, no one was waiting to arrest me at the airport. I caught a train to south Italy and was picked up at the station by the farm manager, Paolo. He had a smile on his face, so my apprehensions began to subside. He shared with me that within two months of starting the vaccination program for brucellosis, there was a sharp decrease in new cases. Actually, there had been no new cases in the last two weeks. Farm owners were pleased and cautiously optimistic. Cattle losses had stopped, and the milk ring test was finally negative for Brucella abortus at the laboratory.

I commented that we would still need to continue the quarterly brucellosis vaccinations and the sanitation measures but it was good to refocus our efforts on profitability instead of Brucella abortus disease losses. From now on, the herd visits could be dedicated to nutrition efficiency, improving reproduction, and improving udder health.

Then Paolo stated that the vaccines were running low and they would have to get more to continue the program. A different method for getting the vaccines had been developed after a frightful experience the first time. In the first shipment, he flew to South America to pick up the medicine, and upon his return to Italy, Paolo was selected by the police to go through the customs inspection line. This had never happened to him before, so he became anxious and perspired heavily as he approached the inspecting officers.

Fortunately, a beautiful young woman was behind him in the line, and the inspector, even after finding the unlabeled bottles in Paolo's luggage, rushed Paolo on through so that he could detain the woman and look through her lingerie. Paolo was sure he would have gone to jail that day if the beautiful woman had not been behind him. The next time vaccine was to be moved they would do it at a time when a friend's relative was working. The relative was employed as a customs agent and could pass them through with the vaccines. This may perhaps have been against the law. It would have been in America!

My friend at the USDA had assured me that the new RB-51 vaccine would not create an immune titer that triggered a positive result in the presently used blood tests. The vaccinations continued for about a year before this assertion was tested. A disgruntled employee reported to officials in northern Italy that the farm was using a strange vaccine, so the northern federal veterinarians conducted a surprise whole herd test. The northern officials did not even tell the southern officials about the testing because they did not trust them (with good reason).

Fortuitously, the surprise test did not reveal a single positive animal. I felt emboldened by this test result and sensed that it was time to share knowledge about this vaccine with a local southern Italy official veterinarian. I did not reveal any of the work in my Italian client's herd, but I did suggest the veterinarian could become somewhat of a hero if he would get the vaccine approved for use in Italy, especially in the buffalo herds. This veterinary official thanked me for the information and later, I found out that he was importing the vaccine himself to sell at an exorbitant price. In time I got out of the RB-51 vaccination business and left it to the Italian "mafia" types.

This disease problem clearly demonstrated the value of the science of epidemiology and the value of disease research. It was a fine example of new technology being applied to an old problem. It was a great example of the roles of a food supply veterinarian keeping the food supply safe, improving animal health, and increasing the production of food through profit.

CHAPTER 38
Heavy Metal Didn't Play Well in Dairies

I was finishing pregnancy testing at a client's dairy in South Carolina when he mentioned that his milk production had recently decreased and his cattle had begun to refuse some of the feed for no apparent reason. This client not only used my reproduction services, but was a nutrition client also. I took a history of recent feeding changes and determined that there were no recent changes. The only feed delivery he had received in the last week was a load of mineral mix from the usual supplier, and it was not a new formula.

To complete my investigation of the production decrease, I walked through and observed the herd, and I sampled the total mixed feed being offered to the cows. When I left the farm, I advised the client that I would immediately mail the sample from a local post office to a trusted commercial feed laboratory, and it would take three days plus shipping time to get the feed analysis results. I promised to telephone him as soon as the results were completed. I was puzzled about the herd production problem because the client had changed nothing, and this producer had always been very meticulous with his adherence to the feeding program.

I worked in South Carolina, a couple more days before I returned to my own dairy farm in North Carolina. The production at my farm had also decreased slightly and there was one cow that my milkmen had concerns about and had separated her away from the herd into a hospital pen. I examined this cow which was unable to rise at this point. Because she was recently calved, I decided to treat her for milk fever or hypocalcimia. I gave the cow an intravenous drip of calcium to try to help her rise, but she was unresponsive. I walked through the herd and observed the cows but noticed nothing remarkable. I pulled samples of my total mixed feed from the feed troughs and mailed them to the same trusted feed laboratory. I was puzzled because I did the nutrition work at my farm and the ration and ingredients had remained the same for months.

The next morning, my down cow was found dead. I loaded her body on a truck and sent it to the state diagnostic laboratory for an autopsy. One of my employees had to transport the cow because I received an emergency call to another client's farm and needed to travel there. Oddly, I began to wonder if the problems at my farm were related to those at the dairy in South Carolina.

When I arrived at the site of the emergency call, I found my dairy client trying to treat two down cows with intravenous calcium. While helping him with this, I began my history-taking process. The notable finding was that these two cows were not recent calvers and should not have gone down with parturient paresis (milk fever). The history also revealed a sudden decrease in milk production and some total mixed feed refusal. I once again walked through and observed the herd. This time I noticed that the cows had some diarrhea, and there was some blood present in the feces.

I pulled some samples of fresh manure and took blood samples from a few of the cows with diarrhea. I also pulled total mixed feed samples from the feed troughs because I also did the nutrition work at this farm. Before I left the farm, one of the down cows we had treated died. I helped load her body on a truck so the dairy client could quickly transport it to the state diagnostic laboratory for an autopsy. On the drive home, I dropped the feed samples off for mailing at a local post office and made my way back to my farm where I had access to a computer. Strangely, I now felt sure there was some relationship between the problems at these three dairies, even though it was improbable. I was the only common thread running through all these farms.

I sat down at my computer and quickly looked up the website for the trusted commercial feed laboratory and downloaded the preliminary report on the feed analysis from the South Carolina dairy. There it was—a heavy metal excess! Because I did the nutrition work, I knew the feed specifications on all these farms and the analysis results contained the first clue to the herd problems. The preliminary analysis showed a lower calcium and a dangerously higher zinc than prescribed specifications. I needed more confirmation before I could definitively diagnose the cause so I quickly left my farm and drove to the state diagnostic lab.

There I logged in my other samples and spoke to the veterinarians involved with the autopsies of the two deceased cows that had been delivered that day. I specifically asked that the lab urgently rush the liver and kidneys to the University of Pennsylvania for testing of zinc, copper and other heavy metal toxins. The North Carolina laboratory did not have the capability for those tests at that time. The reason there was such urgency in the request was this all occurred at the beginning of Thanksgiving week!

These farms were located hundreds of miles apart and grew their own forages. They bought their feed grains from different suppliers. The only commonality on all these farms was me and the company that produced my prescribed, custom vitamin and mineral mixes. I telephoned the manager of the mineral company, whom I knew personally and had worked with for decades, to appraise him of the situation.

He seemed concerned, but he doubted there was a problem because it is very difficult to properly analyze minerals. Their company chemists would check all of this out after the Thanksgiving break in their own special labs. I told him I was nervous about waiting until after Thanksgiving because I was unsure how many of my clients would eventually be affected, and I had already begun to see animal deaths. He assured me there was nothing he could do until after the holidays. This was the Tuesday before Thanksgiving Thursday.

The state diagnostic laboratory reported that they had not found anything in the autopsies to pinpoint a cause of the deaths. This was not unusual with sudden deaths that were not caused by infectious diseases. However, as requested, they had shipped the kidney and liver tissues to Pennsylvania by overnight delivery. On Wednesday evening, I received an email from the diagnostic laboratory at the University of Pennsylvania. The livers and kidneys of both autopsied cows contained toxic levels of the heavy metal zinc.

I had my proof that cows from two different farms died from zinc toxicosis. That night I contacted all three farms and told them to stop using the vitamin mineral mixes from my source company until further notice. The next day on Thanksgiving I telephoned the mineral company manager at home and ruined his holiday. I told him that he could do whatever he wished with his chemists, but I had toxicology from tissues of two cows from different herds showing zinc toxicosis.

Both he and I were baffled about how this could happen—that multiple farms with different mineral prescriptions could be affected by toxic levels of zinc. Both of us suspected a mixing error and not a formulation error because the mineral formulas had been unchanged for many months.

In typical mineral mixes there are macro minerals included at high levels and there are trace minerals included at trace amounts. Zinc is a trace mineral to be fed only in trace amounts because high levels are toxic. I pointed out that the zinc levels in the suspect mineral mixes mimicked the higher levels of the macro minerals instead of the trace levels. The mill manager immediately began an investigation at the mineral company. By Monday, I received the feed analysis reports from my trusted feed laboratory, and all of the total mixed feeds from all of the affected dairies contained excess zinc. I telephoned the mineral company manager and gave him this update. He arranged an emergency meeting with company executives and attorneys.

The story could have ended right here except that I needed to understand the particulars of the problem. I needed to recover some monetary damages for an unknown number of my nutrition clients, and I also needed to be able to trust the mineral company to not have another such occurrence. The mineral company attorneys assured me that they would immediately compensate any of my clients with my calculated damages if there was no litigation initiated. I was satisfied with this assertion.

Then, the mineral plant manager shared the details of what had caused the mixing errors. The company had hired a contractor to make some repairs and upgrades to the distribution head on the tower elevator at the plant. It appeared that this contractor had left some bolts loose on the tower head so that the distributor did not accurately direct mineral ingredients into the correct holding tanks as indicated by the controls of the distributor.

A month before the client's suspect mineral mixes were made, they received and unloaded an entire train carload of zinc sulfate. During the unloading process, some of the zinc went into the calcium holding tank in error. It took some time to use the calcium in the bottom of the tank, and when it was gone, they unknowingly began adding zinc to the mineral mixes at macro levels thinking it to be calcium. With the faulty tower repairs corrected, the distributor was now operating properly.

I was convinced that this problem would not happen again, and the company thanked me for finding the problem so quickly avoiding a sure disaster. All of the mineral mixes for my clients and dozens of other customers, including beef and swine growers, were recalled and replaced. My clients were compensated for their losses which were limited to just a few cows and some minor milk losses at all but one herd. The farm with the greatest losses got a substantial payment and decided to sell his cows and exit the dairy business. "Heavy metal didn't play well at this dairy."

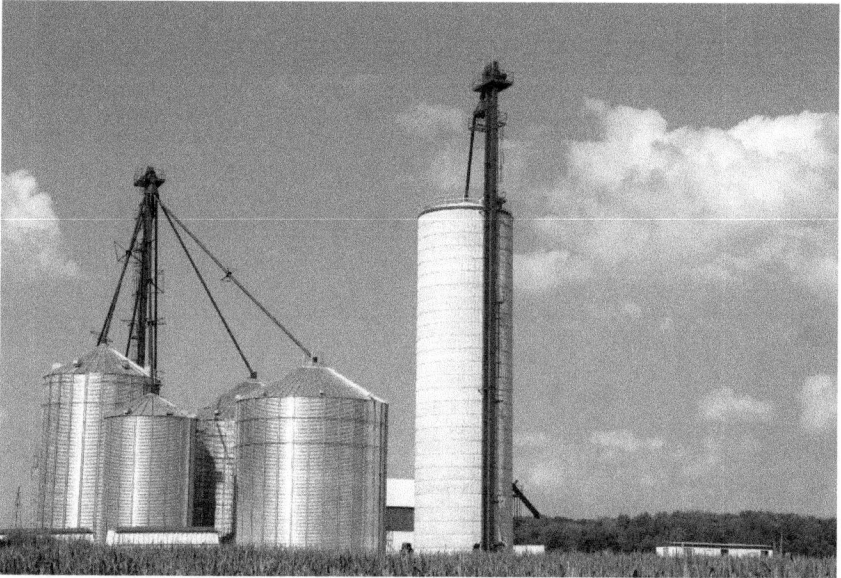

Photo of Feed Mill with Tower Elevator and Distributor Head

CHAPTER 39
Lepto Hardjo—New/Old Problem

For many years in practice I encountered the problem of low fertility in cattle herds. To determine the causes of the infertility I did much testing. I tested blood for diseases. I tested feeds and water for toxins. I evaluated artificial insemination technique and evaluated hundreds of breeding bulls. Sometimes I found an answer that satisfied me and allowed me to make a positive change, but many times I could find no good explanation for the infertility or the cause was yet to be discovered. I was constantly reading research in the cattle reproduction field and attending continuing education conferences because my clients deserved a well-informed clinician.

I frequently suspected the cause of infertility was a group of bacteria called Leptospira. Leptospirosis is the most widespread zoonosis worldwide, causing severe effects on beef and dairy cattle farming and other livestock and sometimes people. Occasionally I could find immune titers to a Leptospira variety such as in chapter 8, "*Buying a Problem*" but, more often, there were no immune titers high enough to definitively diagnose the cause. I often resorted to multiple vaccinations for the disease and maintained them on a quarterly schedule. This approach quite often improved the problem but it was difficult to justify.

Then at the turn of the 20th century a group of veterinarians and scientists in the western United States uncovered an organism called Leptospira hardjo-bovis which seemed to be the culprit in much cattle herd infertility. The naming for this group of organisms is complicated so I will not go into the various Leptospirosis strains or serovars. Suffice it to say that hardjo-bovis is how it is commonly referred to. The scientists that uncovered hardjo-bovis found it not by the common immune blood titer assays, but by examining the urine for live organisms.

The hardjo-bovis serotype is called "host adapted" because it does not stimulate much of an immune response or immune titer. It establishes itself in the kidney tubules where it can continuously contaminate the environment when the animal voids. This bacteria effectively hid from investigators for decades. We veterinarians routinely vaccinated for the five most common Lepto serovars but, because we never knew about Lepto hardjo-bovis, we never vaccinated for the most common cause of bovine infertility.

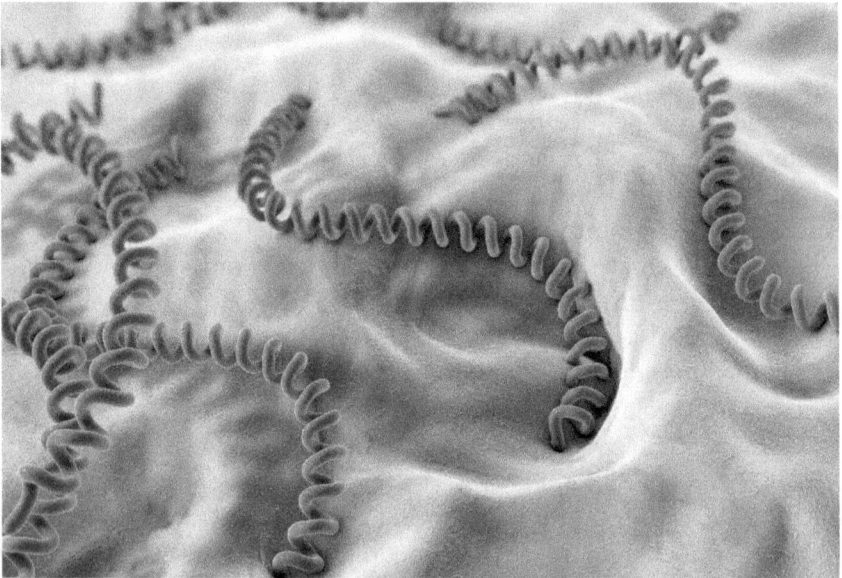

Photo of Leptospira organism in urine under a dark-field microscope.

When I heard about the newly uncovered serovar, I called the vaccine company that was publishing the most data on it. Unfortunately, the new vaccine was being made in Australia and was in short supply. The vaccine company had the policy that a herd would have to be tested positive for the hardjo-bovis disease before they would supply the vaccine to the herd. I obtained detailed instructions on testing and began to test my client herds experiencing infertility.

The testing procedure was challenging and costly. One had to catch a clean sample of the second stream of urine voided after a cow was given an intravenously injected diuretic. At least 10 to 15 percent of the herd needed to be sampled, and immediately afterward, the samples were to be put in dry ice for overnight shipment to a lab in

Michigan.

I tested many of my client's herds. It was rather comical to other people observing, as I followed cows around with a cup on a stick. Nevertheless, I found that 50 percent of the sampled cows in 90 percent of the herds were positive for the live organism in the urine. I eventually vaccinated all of my client herds. The vaccine was very effective, so many of my herds realized a profitable increase in fertility.

As a result of all my testing experience, I became very proficient at testing, and the vaccine company hired me to go to other states in the southeastern United States and survey herds for the disease. The company used my data in their vaccine marketing programs. You should remember that reproduction is the source of all income and resulting profits in food animal agriculture. An important role for food supply veterinarians is increasing the fertility of livestock.

CHAPTER 40
Faith Gives Us Purpose

My senses tell me that the world exhibits intelligent design, put into existence by an intelligent Creator. Therefore, I have faith that there is a higher power known as God. To a Christian, God exists as an amalgamation of the Father, Son, and Spirit. As a person of faith, I believe we all are created for a purpose. I also believe it is important to actively build up and practice our faith. Since I am not a trained religious teacher, I will stop here and get along with the writing of this book.

For over 25 years, I have volunteered with a faith-based mission agency named Christian Veterinary Mission (CVM). Most religiously unreached (or untold) people live in rural or nomadic communities where livestock play a central role in their physical well-being by providing income, nutrition, transportation, clothing, and labor. When these animals are in poor health, are weak, are plagued with disease, or die, it drastically impacts the lives of their owners. Healthy animals can literally make a difference between life and death for an entire family and are often the source of family financial security. CVM leverages its animal knowledge to get invited into these animal-dependent communities to provide training in basic animal husbandry and health care. While CVM volunteers are assisting with physical needs they find opportunities to address spiritual needs. Fortunately, there are many volunteers, including practicing veterinarians, veterinary students, technicians, and family members, who work with CVM and find purpose for their lives in the mission and ministry of Christian Veterinary Mission.

I began my work with CVM by way of a solo mission visit to Santa Cruz, Bolivia. Needless to say it was a pivotal time in my life and greatly strengthened my faith. I was drawn to do this mission by a previous veterinary practice partner Dr. Jim who had gone into full-time mission work after a very selfish prior life. Up until that time, I had never met anyone with such a selfish lifestyle.

Dr. Jim was with his third wife when I met him at our practice. He had left his other two wives and children. He even left this current wife about six months after I arrived, when he left our practice and moved to another job and another woman. Jim had alcohol abuse problems, and I later found out that he also abused drugs. He was judgmental and egotistical and argued readily, especially when drinking. I never wanted to get to know him and was actually glad when he left North Carolina because we were on a personality collision course.

Several years after Jim moved away I had a client approach me about finishing some work Jim had started and not completed because he had given up practice and gone into the foreign missions. All I could say was, "Yeah, right. And, I have some ocean-front property for sale in Arizona." In other words, I did not believe he was capable off mission work. Then, one day as I was perusing a magazine published by CVM, I saw Jim's face in a photo taken while on mission in Bolivia.

I was so overwhelmed with the change he had gone through that I felt compelled to contact him. I called Christian Veterinary Mission's headquarters in Seattle, Washington, and got Jim's email address. I sent him an email saying how proud I was with what he had done with his life, and he sent a reply that he had done nothing—God alone had changed him. This response convinced me that he had truly changed.

Eventually, we were able to speak over the internet through Skype. His voice sounded the same, but his words were humble and kind. The change that had taken place in his worldview was truly amazing, and I began to seek God for a similar change in my life. Jim and I stayed in touch and finally talked on a regular phone during a furlough back to the U.S. He asked me if I would travel to Bolivia and help advise CVM on some of the projects there.

Before I could decide, he and his fifth wife, Randy, both discovered that their parents were ill, and they needed to return to the U.S. Since Jim would not be there and I had heard nothing from CVM, I emailed Jim that perhaps I should wait to travel to Bolivia until after he returned. My real agenda was a longing to see him and feel the faith fire he had in his heart.

However, Jim's agenda was God's agenda. Jim jumped into action, and almost immediately, I received emails from CVM and Phil Bender, the director of the Latin America ministry. My approval for the mission shuttle was granted before the people selected for writing my "required" letters of recommendation had even mailed their evaluations. I also received a package containing advice to help prepare me for overseas mission work. Jim called and once again asked me to consider the shuttle mission. He said, "Everything is arranged. Now, **you** have to make a decision."

At that time, my prayer life was not very good but I needed help making this decision. So, I began to pray daily for some indication of God's will in this matter. While awaiting an answer, I began to work through the overseas mission preparation advice. According to the instructions, I needed three major things —vaccinations listed on the CDC website, a dental check, and a medical physical exam.

I have been blessed with good health, so much so that I didn't even know the name of a local doctor. I had never been ill enough to go to a general physician since moving to Raleigh 19 years before. I asked Shelley, my wife, to get me a physical appointment, but she refused, saying that I was getting older and I needed to find for myself a physician that I was comfortable with. This seemed reasonable so, I called friends in the church and neighbors for recommendations and began contacting their doctors.

The doctors had no appointments for months, or they didn't take new patients. I even cold-called doctors nearby from the phone directory, but their automated answering machines would not allow me to leave messages. That day I called for three-plus hours but could not get through for a single timely appointment. I never anticipated that it would be so difficult to arrange a doctor's visit. Finally, frustrated, I telephoned my wife's female physician thinking I could get a special favor, but found the doctor's office closed.

I was completely frustrated by this time, so in one last desperate attempt, I selected a physician at random from the yellow pages of a nearby town. The name was that of a foreigner, Dr. Arana, and the person answering the phone spoke with a heavy accent. Nonetheless, I determined that this was only for a physical and if the doctor could see me within a month, I would go. I was completely frustrated by the inability to locate a single other physician who would see me at an acceptable time.

To my disbelief, Dr. Arana was able to see me the very next time I had a free day in my schedule—only five days later. This appointment also caught my wife by surprise and she began to wave her hands rapidly, trying to get me to decline the appointment. I put my hand over the phone and told her that it was only for the physical and I would find another doctor later. I needed closure on the decision to go or not, and secretly I hoped the doctor would find something minor wrong, so I could gracefully decide to postpone the trip to Bolivia!

The day before my appointment I called Dr. Arana's office again because there was never any reminder sent, and I also needed to get directions. While on the phone, I asked if there was anything I should do to prepare for the exam and the receptionist questioned, "Like what?" I responded, "Like fast." She then stated that this would be a good idea! I rapidly began to have little confidence in the usefulness of this physical exam, but I went anyway.

When I arrived for the physical, I expected to find a young foreign doctor, not very experienced. Instead, Dr. Arana was very professionally dressed and gray-haired. He shared that he had practiced in the area for over 28 years. The physical he gave was the most thorough I ever received. He took an extensive medical history and wrote it all down. He examined everything, and all examinations were done by him alone. He also took all appropriate blood samples for testing at a commercial diagnostic lab.

I was impressed by his thorough exam, but not as impressed as I was by his medical history taking and medical curiosity. He asked and recorded (no history checklist form) everything about all family members, diseases, causes of death, my work, where I lived, etc. At the end of the exam, he told me he would leave and let me re-dress. When he returned, I expected him to tell me to pay the receptionist on the way out. But no, he stood in front of the door and would not let me leave. He avowed that he could find nothing wrong with me, and my history indicated that I had not seen a doctor nor had a physical for 20 years.

He asked me, "Why are you here?"

I answered, "For a physical."

He was not satisfied with this answer, so he stated, "A man in good health with no history of an exam in 15 to 20 years does not just decide to have a physical. What is bothering you? You must tell me so I can determine if it is a problem for you."

At this, I told him that I was considering going on a mission shuttle to a developing country and Christian Veterinary Mission asked for the physical. Still skeptical, he asked the location of the shuttle and I told him, "Bolivia, South America."

Looking surprised, he said "That is my home, God bless you. Where will you go in Bolivia?"

I answered, "The Santa Cruz area."

He responded again, "That is my home."

My skin began to crawl up my back as I felt the wind of angels flying behind me. I realized that God had just answered my prayers about participation in the shuttle. The answer was clear: I was to go to Bolivia.

Nonetheless, Dr. Arana was not finished yet. He asked, "Are you having any problems with arrangements?"

I answered that I had difficulty with which vaccines were needed. He then took me across the hallway into his office where there was a laminated poster on the wall entitled "Vaccinations Needed for Santa Cruz, Bolivia." He next called the Health Department and scheduled all appropriate travel vaccinations. Then we returned to the exam room and, once again, he asked if there was anything else of concern.

I don't know why, but I felt compelled to mention my concern over my friend Jim not being there to meet me. In response to this, he reached for his prescription pad, and on the back of it he wrote down the name and telephone number of his best friend in the world, an anesthesiologist in Florida who was retiring the next week. His friend was returning home to Santa Cruz to of all things--- a dairy farm that he owned. Amazingly, I was scheduled to speak at the first annual Bolivian Dairy Symposium while on this mission!

Dr. Arana cautioned me to call right away, and his friend would meet me there. Praise the Lord! Not only had God shown me His will for me, but He opened every door that seemed to be an impediment to the trip. To this day I believe that finding only Dr. Arana available for my physical was not a coincidence—it was Providence!

Over the years, I learned that if you are seeking God, go serve those most in need, and you will find Him there! During this first solo (alone) mission, I saw and experienced many things that broke my heart. There was so much poverty, hunger, abuse, and superstitious darkness. Children were especially subjected to exploitation. Such a hard existence! I knew that if these things broke my heart, then they also broke God's heart. One evening I felt so overwhelmed that in tears, I prayed to God, asking why He would show me all of this suffering at this late time in my life when by myself I could do little to improve the future for these people.

I asked God, "How can I make a difference in their lives?" Amazingly, and also providentially, the answer was clear to me when I awakened the next morning. I was not to go alone on missions in the future. I was to take young veterinary students with me and build in them a heart for service. Learning to listen to God is the most important lesson you will ever learn. In my mind and heart, this revelation was the beginning of the student outreach program at CVM. Thus, for over 25 years, I have been mobilizing young people to serve God and mankind through CVM and their veterinary missions. The following story is from a journal kept on an early mission.

CHAPTER 41
Veterinary Student Mission to Bolivia

Preface: In 2000, I did not intend to return to Bolivia another year in succession. There were some health problems in my family (my health and my mother's), there were many problems in my clients' dairy operations, and my schedule was very full. I also wished that on my next mission trip, I could take my wife, Shelley. However, she felt unable to go in 2000.

Nonetheless, there were other plans in the making. I was called by World Concern in Bolivia requesting another visit. I was called by Christian Veterinary Mission in Seattle, Washington to consider guiding another student shuttle mission. And eventually, I was called by the student Christian Veterinary Mission Fellowship group at North Carolina State University's College of Veterinary Medicine requesting help in organizing a shuttle mission for them.

I began to pray about these requests, and I felt the call of the Lord to do this shuttle mission. God's commanding is God's enabling so I knew that God would provide.

The shuttle mission began by arranging a meeting and a presentation for the students about the previous year's mission. There was great excitement in the student group and a genuine longing to share their skills and love of God in this special way. I was hooked by their excitement and, at the same time, very anxious about my ability to lead a mission team that would meet everyone's expectations. I prayed for guidance, wisdom, and confidence. The shuttle needed to be set for early December to allow for the students to complete their exams. The busy schedule of the students allowed for only one other meeting before departure.

We had dinner and a group prayer at my home to set the tone for the mission. We discussed health regulations, clothing needs, and travel particulars. We agreed to stay in touch through email until after exams. Although the timing of the shuttle was not great for me or my wife, we accepted the needs of the students as God's planning. As it turned out, the early December departure date gave us more time to raise support and donations, and more time to pray for the success of the mission and its projects.

The day before the shuttle group was to leave for Bolivia we found out that there was a box embargo in Bolivia. I had never heard of a box embargo before. We had collected many items for donation in Bolivia that required transport. The shuttle group met to plan alternatives to boxes. We would all take two large suitcase bags and pack the donated materials among our clothes. We tightly packed all of the donated materials into the bags, and every one of the bags was safely checked all the way to Santa Cruz. Praise the Lord! The flights were a little rough but uneventful. We arrived in Santa Cruz, Bolivia on time with all of our bags.

Upon arrival we checked into the Hotel Internacional and went to lunch in the city with one of our hosts. A good three-course meal in Santa Cruz cost our group of 7 plus the host translator only $12.00. After lunch we met with the local World Concern personnel, reviewed our itinerary, and received our arrival briefing.

That night we held our first of many evening devotional meetings. The meetings were important to allow the team to discuss the events and activities of the day and to allow the team members to express their feelings about the impact of the mission on their life outlook (world view) and personal faith journey.

Las Gamas

Our first project was a visit to the Las Gamas women's dairy project. This is a joint Heifer Project International, World Concern, and Bolivian government project for the empowerment of poor women. I had visited this dairy project on previous shuttle missions. These rural women had formed a cooperative to begin a dairy for the support of their families. Each mother had multiple children—beginning motherhood at 15 to 16 years old. I got the impression that most of the fathers were not around any longer. In Bolivia, many "marriages" are common law, and the men often take very little responsibility for the children, and provide little support. There is no legal enforcement and no social safety net for abandoned families.

The extreme poverty cycle continues without the help of projects such as this women's dairy. Along the road to Las Gamas, we saw a new power line made possible by donations from my supporters on last year's mission. I felt proud and excited about being a part of the important improvements in this community. Before the power line the women had to complete all feed processing, watering, and milking of the cows by hand. Now the women had electricity and running water!

At the previous day's World Concern briefing we had been advised that there was concern about a mean cow which calved two weeks ago. She was difficult to milk and restrain, and the women were beginning to fear her. It was critical for the success of this project that the women not fear the animals. At the farm we found the women unafraid. It was the people at the World Concern office who were unfamiliar with cattle that were really afraid.

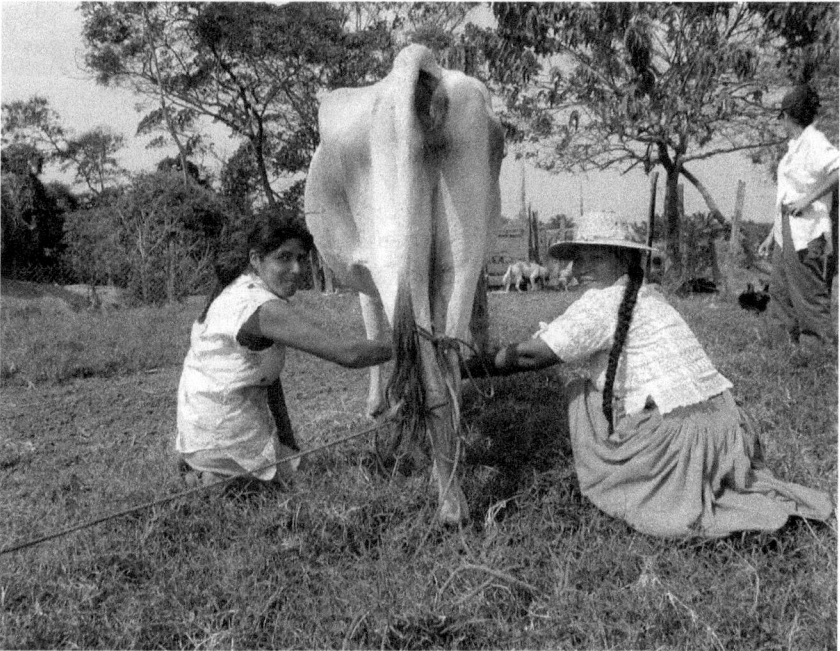

The women of the project first gave us a presentation of the goals of the project and also a presentation of the philosophy of the women in the project. I was impressed with their organization, comprehension, and dedication to this project, to God, and to each other. It was truly a positive change from their attitudes on the previous visit. The women then accompanied us to the new dairy located on a large parcel of land-- quite an impressive facility for Bolivia. The crops were good and the twelve cattle were in good condition. Feeding methods were reviewed and plans were discussed for intensive grazing using an electric fence charger and polywire fencing which our shuttle group had voted to donate to the women's project. I have always tried to make a long lasting gift to mission projects---this year electric fencing, the first year an electric line, another year was irrigation, etc.

Although there was a bull present at the farm the women asked for one cow to be inseminated artificially and the others to be checked for dates of calving. This was done with the help of the women and they handled the cows well. The women had never seen a cow bred artificially so I tried to make a little presentation out of the process. It is interesting to note that the frozen semen for artificial insemination should be thawed in warm water, so I requested a small container of hot water be brought to me. After impatiently waiting for about half an hour, I decided to go see what could be causing the delay and found that two of the women had built a fire to heat the water. I had forgotten where I was when I asked for hot water—such a common commodity in America.

At Las Gamas in addition to working with cattle, we repaired fences, repaired broken water pipes and repaired the water pump. We had a few tools from the World Concern office. The women have no tools. We planned to return the following day to help with some animal handling improvements and to give more help with the intensive grazing project.

We had trouble getting out of Santa Cruz the next day. There was only one driver available so we all had to pile into one little Toyota pickup truck—half of the group in the back. After this trouble, we left late for Las Gamas. The student group was excited about this trip because they enjoyed the first day at Las Gamas so much. They had prepared plans for the intensive grazing project using the electric fencing. They had also brought candy and Bibles for gifts. With half the group in the back of the little truck, we hoped for clear weather. At Las Gamas we were rebuked for our late arrival, not for tardiness because this is Bolivia, but because the women were afraid we were not coming.

The women began by giving all of us gifts. It was very moving because they made the gifts by hand and can afford so little. After a quick lunch we went to the dairy on foot. There was a great deal of bonding that occurred during the walk to the dairy. The students now have been touched as deeply by these women and their needs as I had been. The students gave their grazing presentation to the women by acting like cows. Everyone enjoyed the "cow play" greatly. It was hard to say goodbye, because many of the students knew they would never see these new friends again. That night we had a discussion of the day's observations. The students responded well. Everyone shared and prayed for the first time. It was apparent that God was touching us and we ended with a group bidding prayer. Tomorrow was Sunday and would be a day of rest and reflection.

Yappacani

Monday we awoke at 6 a.m. to go to the Yappacani region. The first half of the day was spent in travel and meetings with officials, farmers, and veterinarians to teach them about the diseases of human tuberculosis (TB) and the zoonotic disease, bovine (cow) tuberculosis (TB). We, Christian Veterinary Mission, had agreed to begin a nationwide cattle testing program designed to determine if the regional dairy industry played a part in the human TB problem in Bolivia. This region of Bolivia had the highest incidence of human TB in the Western Hemisphere and was the perfect place to start the program.

Bolivia did not have the funds to do the testing themselves, so Christian Veterinary Mission arranged to provide help. There was great resistance to the proposed testing program because of the potential for the government destroying affected animals. The farmers were reluctant, even though there was a risk to cattle and people from TB, because the cattle are their major means of economic support. I met with the reluctant farmer groups and explained through an interpreter the importance of finding and removing positive animals as a future requirement for keeping their market for meat and milk. I explained that I had examined the human records and found the TB to be of the lung type and not the digestive type characteristic of bovine TB.

Therefore, I explained that I expected to find very little cattle tuberculosis if any at all. I also suggested that they organize into a cooperative that helps reimburse the farms that must destroy animals. This way, all farms would submit to testing and the region's cattle population could be certified free, to preserve the market by demonstrating the safety of the food supply. With this final suggestion and after much discussion, they all agreed to test for TB.

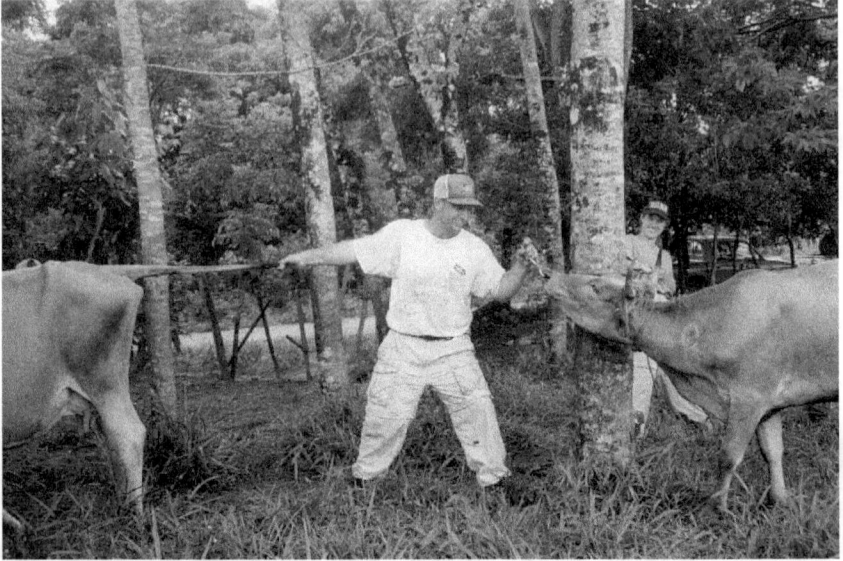

In the afternoon, we went into the countryside, which was really the Amazon jungle, to do a comparative TB test on a few animals. The area was beautiful, but the roads were terrible. We had to ford one river and several creeks. It took two hours to reach the farthest farm before we could work our way back. No surprise there were no cattle handling facilities. We were required to rope the animals and tie them to a tree or cast them on the ground to perform the tests. Needless to say, this resulted in quite a rodeo with the resistant subjects.

Fortunately no one was hurt during the process. We finished about 9 p.m. in the dark. We ate crackers and bananas for supper that we had bought that morning in Santa Cruz. I was reluctant to expose the team to restaurants in this remote area because of sanitation concerns. Plans were made to purchase much of our food and all of our water for the return to this area later in the week. We arrived in Santa Cruz very tired at midnight. The day felt successful since the program to begin TB testing was accepted. Our goal when we returned to the area was to test 400 to 800 animals. This is quite a goal with the primitive methods available. Each evening we gathered and discussed the day. This evening was a short meeting. We prayed for our safety, and success in the week, and for our families back home.

We rose and departed Santa Cruz at 6 a.m. the next morning. The first stop was the World Concern office where we gathered all equipment and luggage needed for six days in Yappacani. We put tarps on the equipment in the backs of the trucks in case of rain, because this was the rainy season in Bolivia. Little did we know that it would rain every day in Yappacani. Our last stop on the road out of town was at the grocery store to buy food and water for one to two meals each day. This would reduce expenses and reduce exposure to potentially dangerous food in the remote areas.

We arrived in the rain at Yappacani and went to the Hotel Turista, our home for the next six days and nights. Then we went to a restaurant of sorts. It was outdoors with a grass roof, but the floor was concrete. I cautioned everyone to eat only the cooked, hot foods or fruits they could peel at the table. These precautions came from my days in the military where I served as the food safety officer on base. This restaurant's standard fare was hot soup every day, even in 90-degree weather, followed by fried yucca, fried bananas, rice, and meat, and the food started to taste good by the end of the week. I had great concern for the health of the group during this week because sanitation was minimal in this remote place. Fortunately, everyone made it through the week with only minor digestive upsets by following proper eating precautions.

After lunch, we broke into two teams. The local veterinarian was with team 1, and I was with team 2. Team 1 had two vaqueros (cowboys), and we had a vet student from Santa Cruz and one vaquero. My team returned to read the TB tests begun three days before, and team 1 began testing new cattle. Team 1 really enjoyed their afternoon. There was no rain, and they left the road hiking to three farms of 15 to 20 cows each. The scenery for them was spectacular. Each farm had a small corral, and things progressed well. The only complaint was they did not take water on this four-hour trek because no one could tell them in English that they would be away from the truck all afternoon.

My group, team 2, didn't do so well. We had only a few cows from six farms eligible to read TB tests. Two farms never got the cattle up, and at two other farms we could only capture one-half of the subjects. I made the decision to stop chasing and hunting cows and to return to the other group after one cow escaped and members of the group chased her for one to two miles over the hilly jungle terrain. The last time we saw her, she and her calf were disappearing over a ridge three hills distant from us. We all returned to the hotel and cleaned up for supper. We went to the vaquero restaurant and had some tough beef alongside some rice with local cheese mixed in. This food did not settle well.

We found out that the town of Yappacani doesn't care whether it's day or night. It's always bustling if the sky is clear. That first night was clear, so the dogs and chickens and people made a racket all night. I didn't sleep much at all. When it rains the town gets quiet. Yappacani reminds me of the "Old West" cattle trail towns. It is the only place for hundreds of miles where people can get needed supplies for cooking, farming, and medical needs. All the milk produced in this area comes here for cooling and transport to larger cities. The town has 40,000 residents with over 100,000 people wandering around on most days.

There is only one hotel, Hotel Turista, with eight rooms, so many people sleep in bunkhouses or on the streets. The only paved road is through the center of town, and all the others are mud. Actually, this paved highway is one of the two major paved roads in Bolivia that intersect in Santa Cruz. There are some other short paved segments of roads, but 95 percent of roads in Bolivia are dirt.

I had to take over driving duties for our team the next morning. Only a few of the Bolivians we worked with had any driving experience. Once again, we started at 6 a.m., determined to make more progress than the day before. But, we were met by cloudy skies, and by noon, the rains came in torrents. We tried to finish the herds in which we were working; however, any further work was impossible. The optics in the last herds of the day, when the heavy rains started were quite comical. People had no footing when the cows were lassoed, so the cattle just pulled the vaqueros around, dragging them across the wet grass until they had to let go. We lost only one cow (and rope) in the end, and I believe she is still out about the jungle with our rope.

By 2:00 p.m. we retired to the hotel to eat and wait out the rain, which never stopped until after dark. That night we found a place called "Okey Chicken." After blessing the food and thanking God for our safety, we gorged ourselves on fried chicken, French fried potatoes, fried bananas, and rice. Bolivian chickens are not very smart because they were walking all around our legs during the meal while we ate their fried comrades.

Later the surprise of the evening was the appearance of one of the Bolivian vaqueros with a guitar. We were in the middle of our usual evening devotional session, so we stopped telling cowboy stories and began to sing hymns together. The young vaquero played guitar for his church, so we enjoyed his music and our chance to praise God together. The night was rainy, so dogs, roosters, and people stayed inside and quiet. I slept like a rock.

The next morning we began again at 6 a.m., once again determined to test more cows than the day before. It was again raining torrents and the local veterinarians refused to work. We decided to go ahead. The roads were terrible and the creeks and rivers swollen. Nonetheless, we had a group prayer and erased all obstacles. The rains stopped when we reached the first farms. The day was long and hard but uneventful. We never left the field but ate fruit and crackers between farms. By the end of the day we were rejoined by all our local help, and we tested over 200 cattle. Over all, we had injected over 520 animals.

After Okey Chicken, we went to a local church to meet some Bolivian friends and sang praises again for an hour or so. We got wet again that night walking back to the hotel. By this time, my boots and feet had been wet for three days. My boots wouldn't dry until Sunday—four days later. After evening devotions, we went to bed, and all slept well. It rained all night.

We read TB tests that Friday from Tuesday's injections. Tuesday was the rain-out day, so this day was short. In the early afternoon, we went to a small local university at Yappacani. This university trained the people who worked with us daily. We gave them an internet ready computer that we had brought into Bolivia and donated it to them. They were very appreciative because the computer and modem connected their library to all the libraries in the world.

Everyone on the team appreciated the afternoon rest in preparation for Saturday when we would have to catch over 200 animals for the second time in three days. We washed some clothes and shopped for water and snacks for the full day in the field that awaited us. After Okey Chicken and evening devotions, we retired.

We started early at 6 a.m. again. It rained off and on through the day, so we were once again a little short of help because the Bolivian veterinarians don't work in the rain. This meant that we would have to do some of our own roping. Of course, this led to some comical competition between each other and between us and the cows.

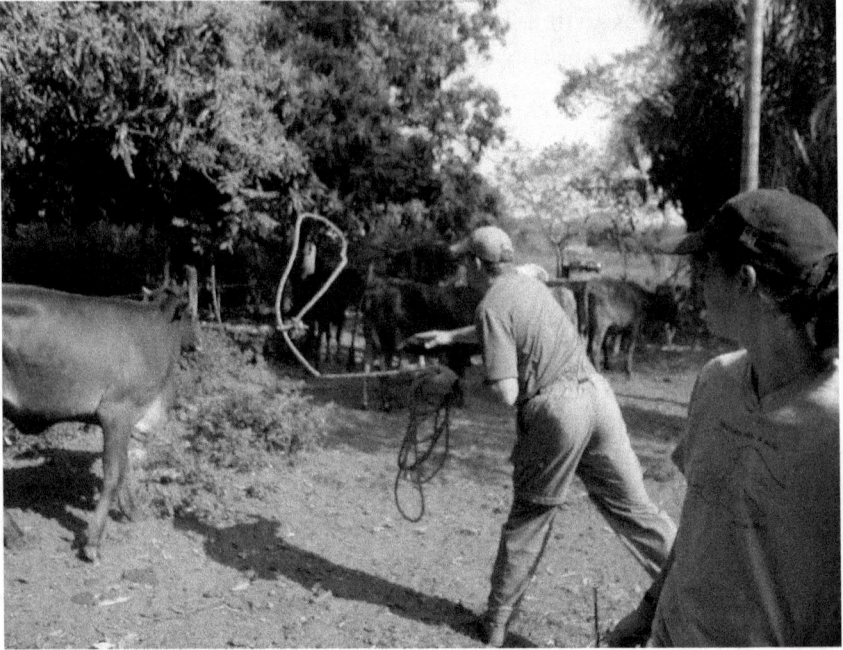

Team 2 finished early, so we drove to join the others and help them finish. The day was successful and uneventful, except when my team's truck died on the highway. We were eventually able to restart it and never found out why it shut down. Perhaps it had something to do with us giving 17 people a lift to town in our little Toyota truck. Every day we gave people rides into town because their only transportation was bicycles or foot. Most can afford only one bicycle, and this is used daily to transport milk toward town, which may be up to 15 miles away as in the example shown on the following page.

That evening we met with the Bolivian technicians who had worked with us during the week. We had brought some veterinary bags for them from the U.S. with various instruments and supplies. We were so touched by their excitement at getting these gifts. These people are well trained but very poor. The doctor kits were beyond their dreams.

The next day we returned to Santa Cruz after packing the trucks with luggage and supplies. It was a beautiful day with sunshine and a breeze. We took this opportunity to tour around the city and shop for our loved ones back home. It was very near Christmas, and for the first time we began to feel the Christmas spirit. It was strange that

Christmas was coming in the middle of the summer here. The city was decorated with many of the same decorations and Santas that we see in the U.S.

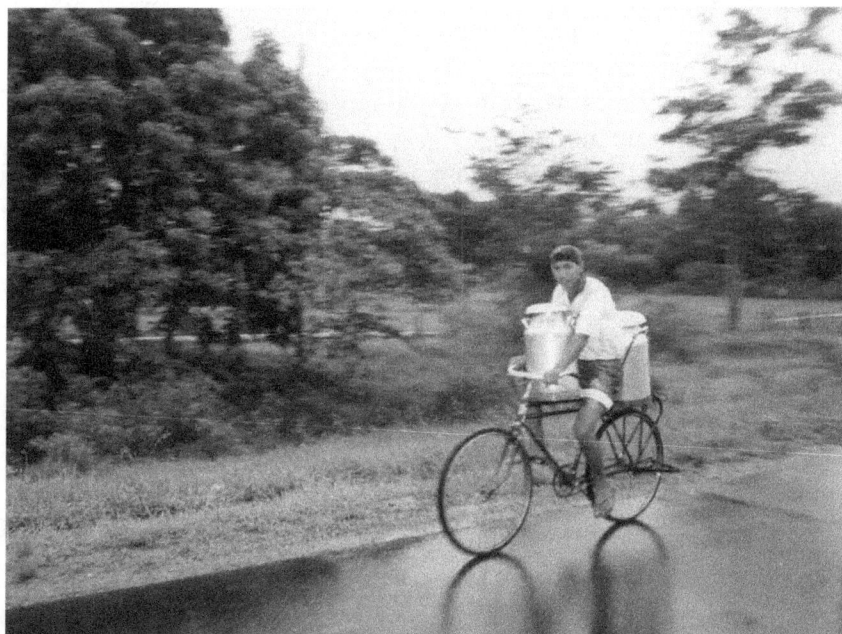

In the evening, during devotions and discussions, we talked about our work and results of the TB testing to prepare for Monday's debriefing. We also talked about home and favorite Christmas traditions with family. We thanked God for His Son and our safety over the last days and asked for safe travel to rejoin our loved ones.

Finally, it was the last full day of the shuttle mission before we flew back to America. Our first task was getting our travel clothes to the laundry. After a week of sweat and rain, everything wreaked. From the laundry, we went to the World Concern office for a formal thank you and debriefing. The results of our work in the Yappacani region showed no positive animals for human or bovine TB. The only positives were to avian (bird) tuberculosis and this is no threat to mammals. The farmers were ecstatic that their market was secure from the health perspective.

We shared with the World Concern personnel additional donations from our mission shuttle supporters to distribute to the people of Bolivia. There were donations of about $2000 worth of cattle dewormers from pharmaceutical companies that went into the supplies of World Concern for resale to poor farmers at discounted prices. There were also many Spanish Bibles and children's books. The Bibles and books were donated from churches in America. Some Bibles and books were given to the women and children at the Las Gamas women's dairy, some were given to World Concern to be used in various communities where needed, and some were taken to a local orphanage by our shuttle team.

The visit to the orphanage was special. This orphanage had 27 children and was very well run with six volunteers and two permanent staff. All of them were from outside of Bolivia, and they loved the children very much. Most of the volunteers were young college-age men and women who gave at least one year of their life to the orphanage.

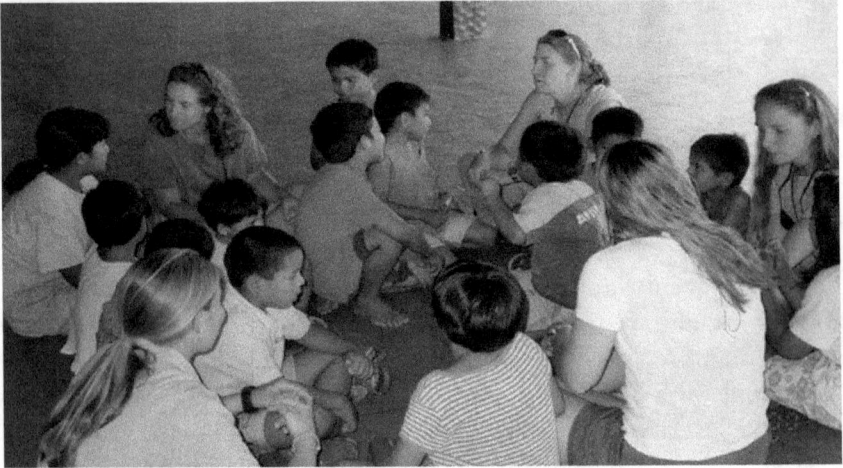

The Vet Students at the Orphanage.

We had pizza as our last evening meal in Bolivia with the Latin-American World Concern director and his family. After pizza, we went into the downtown area to have ice cream at McDonalds. We were beginning our re-entry into U.S. culture. While downtown, however, we were surrounded by little children begging for money. This was a constant occurrence, but tonight it made a more profound impression. During the evening devotions and discussions, we talked about the street children and their homeless mothers. These are the real tragedies in Bolivia. The orphaned children had food, warmth, love, and many opportunities. The children of Yappacani were very poor, but they had two parents, love, food, and a primitive home. The street children in the city are truly the disenfranchised population in Bolivia, and our only solution for them at this point in the shuttle was prayer. We have faith that conditions will improve for these little ones.

We were given the opportunity to lead the devotions for the whole World Concern office through an interpreter. The witness and testimonies by the group were almost too much for me. What better way to grow your faith than by working side by side with someone who is hurting or has needs greater than yours? I realized that God had truly touched each of us and blessed us through this opportunity to help the people of Bolivia through Christian Veterinary Mission. We were all given gifts by the World Concern team as tokens of their thanks.

Then, lastly, they gave me a plaque naming me an honorary member of the World Concern Bolivia team. I tried desperately to keep my composure, but nonetheless, got choked up. I could have received no greater compliment than to be considered a part of this dedicated group of Christian missionaries. We were truly partners in their mission, and the relationships we established were deep and lasting. This was the mission God had sent us to accomplish.

From the various mission shuttles that I made to Bolivia, four participants went into full-time mission service. Two returned to work in Bolivia, and two are serving in India. Over the years, I have led numerous shuttle missions to the Native Americans, Kenya, Costa Rica, and Mexico, and there have been hundreds of participants given access to faith-building mission activities. Many of the participants on these shuttles also committed to further service through CVM and other mission agencies.

The revelation given to me on my first mission trip of "do not go alone" has given me years of fruitful purpose and has sustained my faith. As a food supply veterinarian, I was truly blessed that God would use my passion for wholesomely feeding people to advance His Kingdom. Indeed, this book would probably never have been written if it were not for the encouragement of the students on these shuttle missions, who constantly cajoled me to write these stories down after I would share them in our small group settings. These students that I thought I was mentoring were actually mentoring and ministering to me.

CHAPTER 42
Veterinary Student Missions to the Navajo

After several years of missions to Bolivia, the populace in Bolivia elected a coca (cocaine) producer as president of the country. With the change in national leadership the security of the student teams became questionable, so I worked out with CVM to begin shuttle missions to the Native Americans.

The Navajo are the largest Native American tribe in the United States, so they were chosen for the earliest mission shuttles. From these early shuttles I identified a special young Christian veterinarian named Dr. Page Wages who had a real heart for the Native Americans. Dr. Page and I made over 20 annual trips to the Navajo and eventually she took over as the mission leader. Before she assumed leadership we both realized that few students had a valid concept of what mission service entailed and even fewer "easterners" understood the world of the Native Americans.

As a result we began offering a course at the veterinary college aptly called Missions Preparedness Class. The class which taught about missions and the Navajo culture was a hit with the students and has continued to be taught for more than a decade. Over the years we have shared with the students what our goals for the mission shuttles were. The goals were broken down into Major Goals and Minor Goals and are listed below:

Major Goals of Mission

- Build the faith of participants
- Spread the Gospel to those in need
- Fellowship with and build up other Christians

- Improve the condition of people and animals
- Improve the skills of veterinary students
- Build in the participants a heart for service

Minor Goals of Mission

- See and appreciate the awesomeness of God's creation
- Learn to work on a team
- Develop skills in evangelism
- Learn to organize and complete a mission project
- Learn to raise support –prayers and financial
- Develop opportunities to share the mission experiences

Each mission team and mission shuttle had its own character. This is what piqued the interest of the leaders making the mission activity so much fun and so inspirational year after year. Each year more and more students joined us on the Navajo mission. We began with a group of seven and maxed out at over 22. Hundreds of dedicated young missionaries have participated. Every year we would drive out to save funds and to be able to carry all of our medical supplies. The trip was 2400 miles one way, taking about 36 hours.

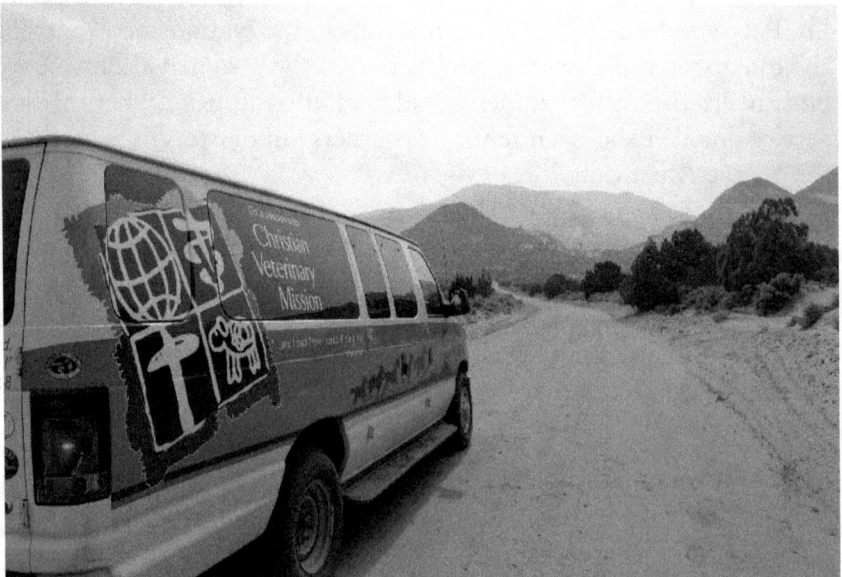

Dr. Page's van with Navajo Mountain in the background.

When 15 passenger rental vans became scarce, Dr. Page personally purchased two of them and had them wrapped in Christian Veterinary Mission logos. She was devoted to CVM and the Native Americans, and was in God's will on the missions. During the 20-plus years of successive annual mission trips we met so many awesome people among the student missionaries, and also, residing in the Navajo Nation. It quickly became apparent that the most important part of these missions was not the veterinary work we accomplished but the relationships we built. I could never have imagined the special way that God would bless and use me years ago when I entered Dr. Arana's exam room. The following notes are from mission shuttles to the Navajo during the first decade of the 21st century.

2001

One of the first impactful people we met was **Kent Greymountain**. Kent worked as a livestock agent for the Navajo Nation at Tuba City, Arizona and as a grazing official at Navajo Mountain, Utah. He spent many days with us during each shuttle mission, especially the first several years of Navajo trips. Kent had so much patience with the teams and all of their questions and criticisms. He explained the Navajo culture, the attitudes of the Navajo toward "Anglos", including the reasons for distrust of "Anglos" after years of oppression and injustice.

Kent also introduced us to most of the other extraordinary people we grew to love over the ensuing years; the people that inspired us and made our trips such special events. Kent was responsible for taking us to the Navajo Mountain area and introducing us to his own family there. Navajo Mountain became the most special place during the missions; because it is the most remote area of the Navajo Nation and there is an annual celebration called "Pioneer Day" each August. We made sure the trip dates included the first Saturday in August so we could see all our friends at "Pioneer Day."

Mrs. Stella Drake and her family were special friends and mentors to our mission teams from the first visit. Stella was quite a character, well-educated and well-traveled (traveled to Paris!), but chose to live at Navajo Mountain. Her husband Henry Drake founded the "Pioneer Day" celebrations when he was serving on the Navajo Tribal Council, the Nation's main governing body. Actually, "Pioneer Day" is the "Anglo" term for *Naa Tsis aan Eehaniih*, which is the Navajo phrase for

"Celebration of the Old Ones". This celebration commemorates the clever old Navajo who resisted capture by the U.S. Cavalry and hid in the Navajo Mountain area for years while the majority of the tribe was incarcerated at Fort Sumner, New Mexico. The following photo is in memory of Mrs. Stella Drake.

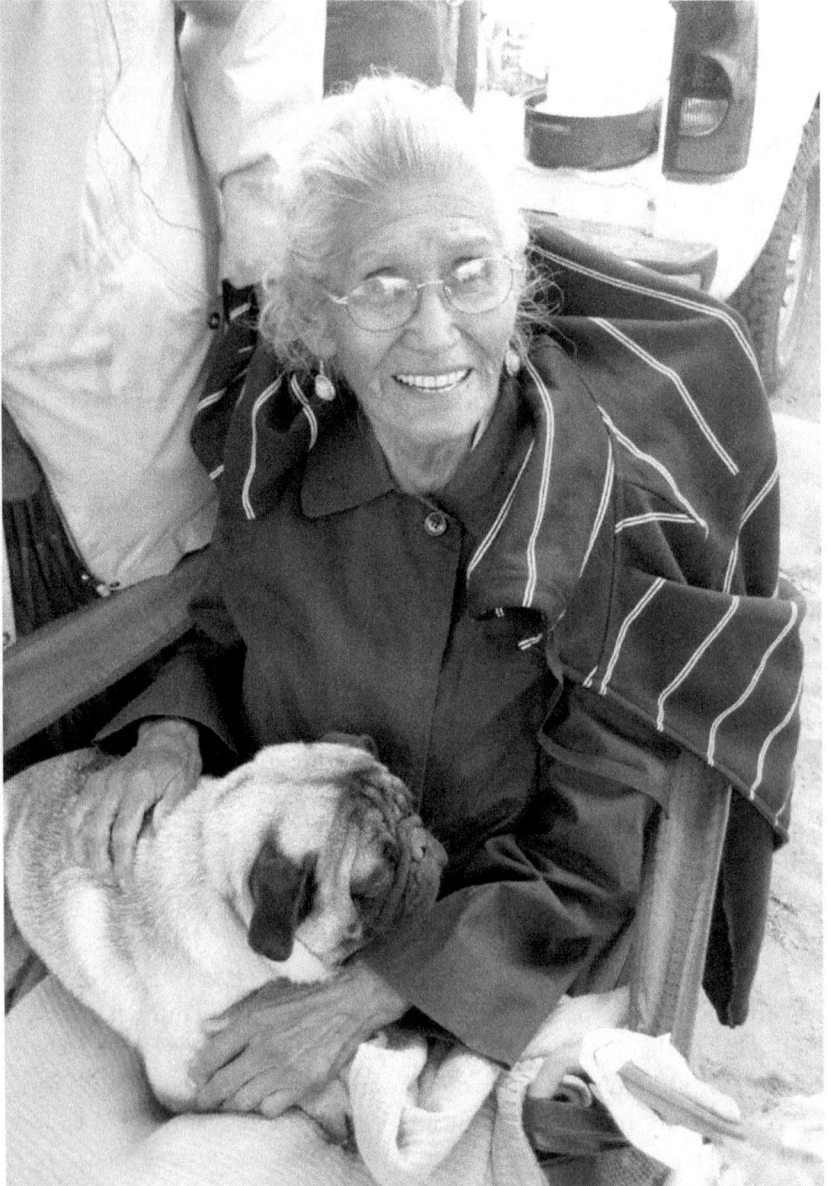

Stella Drake with her favorite pet.

Stella explained that the Navajo were forced to march to Fort Sumner from their homes all over the Navajo Nation in a march called the "Long Walk." The tribe was allowed to return four years later after they signed treaties they could not read. However, many of the elders did not survive this treatment, so the tribe was left without the knowledge to survive in the arid land. Nevertheless, when the "Old Ones" who had escaped capture heard that the Dine' (the people) had returned, they quickly intercepted them and taught them the skills they needed to survive to this era.

Lucky for us, Stella spoke perfect English and was such a wonderful storyteller. The team made every effort to gather at her house each night so we could sit and hear her stories. She also shared her Navajo cooking skills with every team, teaching each to make the delicious Navajo Taco. Stella was a strong Christian woman and one of my fondest memories is of singing "Jesus Loves Me" together with her family. They sang in Navajo and we sang in English. Stella has now gone to see the Lord, but her family still travels to Navajo Mountain each year for Pioneer Day where we reunite with them and celebrate the "Old Ones."

We have another special connection with Drake family. Stella's granddaughter, Tara, aspired to be a veterinarian after joining us at Navajo Mountain during our shuttle missions. She loved the animal work we did and what we stood for. She participated with our teams year after year as a teenager until as a young woman she applied for veterinary college. When she applied for veterinary school we had the privilege to write recommendations for her. She was accepted to vet school and missed a few shuttle missions, but this past year she joined us again as a graduate veterinarian!

2002

Our mission team was honored to be given a task at Pioneer Day this year. Many of the Navajo people walked or rode horses to the celebration, just as their ancestors had done. The whole weekend was one big family fair, the Navajo way. They loved competitions of all kinds. There were horse races, foot races, tug-o-wars, and sprints to pick up prizes. The children, ran for toys and stuffed animals, the young married men sprinted for cooking pots, and even the elder ladies sprinted and ran for purses secretly holding money or amusement park tickets.

We were assigned the duty of laying out toys on the parade ground for the competitions. To us this job was so special; to be included in this important Navajo celebration. Unexpectedly, at noon we were asked to clear the parade ground for the honoring of the Navajo military veterans and for the presentation of the nation's colors. Astonishingly, 30 percent the Navajo people serve in the U.S. military. Compare that to less than five percent for Americans. I was impressed with the appearance of dozens of veterans in full uniform from many of our nation's wars and conflicts. The head of ceremonies read the names of those present and lavished praise on our United States. He extolled their pride in serving and their willingness to give their lives for America. They even sang the National anthem in Navajo and English.

I could not believe what I was hearing! This Dine' Nation had forgiven America for taking everything from them and parking them on this reservation. They had forgiven the oppression and injustice and fully embraced the principles of the United States despite the past. I could not control my emotions and wept uncontrollably. This happened many years in succession.

Over the years we provided animal health services to many of the Navajo families, and gracefully they showed their appreciation by introducing us as the "Christian Veterinarians" before the whole Pioneer Day crowd and giving handmade Native Navajo gifts to us individually. Following is the presentation of the colors.

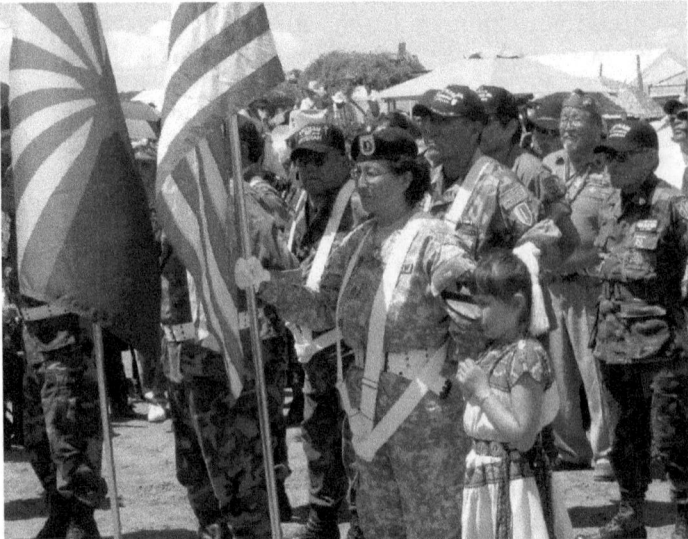

2003

This year, we met the **"Little" family**—Berna, Tim, and Ron. Berna had been an important person in the Navajo culture because she was a medicine woman. She lived on Navajo Mountain and gave all of this power up when she became a Christian after being taught by a traveling Native American preacher. Berna resolutely determined to raise her sons Tim and Ron as Christians, despite the persecution and oppression from her family and friends. Legend has it that Berna's husband was very opposed to her Christian life and was one of the worst oppressors. He challenged her that unless her God returned a four-month missing horse (which he believed was dead), he would never accompany her to church at the base of the mountain.

Berna prayed fervently, and the next morning the horse was standing outside the door of their hogan (home). The husband went with the family to church the next Sunday. Berna never verified this story to me because she only spoke Navajo. Nonetheless, the sons became strong Christians and were mentors of our teams for many years. Tim came to our evening devotions, and Ron often procured horses for members of our group to ride to Pioneer Day with the Navajo riders. What an authentic, surreal experience!

Most years, we vetted the "Little" family's cattle; however, every year, we vaccinated and dewormed Berna's sheep and goats. Berna loved us because we were fellow Christians and because we cared for her herd. Every year, she handmade gifts for us as a reward for returning to the Navajo people and taking care of their animals. To the traditional Navajo, the small ruminants were their most prized assets, their bank accounts, and their retirement funds.

The outside world looks at the poverty in the Navajo Nation—the lack of jobs, the many people without electricity and running water, the inability to borrow money to build housing, not being able to own their land—and they wonder how these people survive. Traditional Navajo have existed for generations solely on these small herds of animals. The small ruminants are the real survivors, and with the protection of the Navajo herdspersons, they helped the Navajo survive. Berna not only understood this, she lived it. She and I formed a special bond through her animals. We never had a conversation, but every time I went to the Navajo Nation I worked with her herd and found her, and prayed with her—each in our own native language. Berna has now joined her ancestors and her Lord.

Berna and her family taught us about the traditional Navajo religion. To summarize, the Native Americans worshiped the world they lived in. She and her family chose to worship the Creator of that world. She explained this so well through her sons that Dr. Page and I wrote an article entitled "Serving the Creator, Not the Created" which was published in a national magazine. Her picture graces the article and her wisdom is her legacy. Berna touched me and honored me by gifting me with her own personal turquoise necklace that she wore daily. I have memorialized this gift by using it in my internet profile.

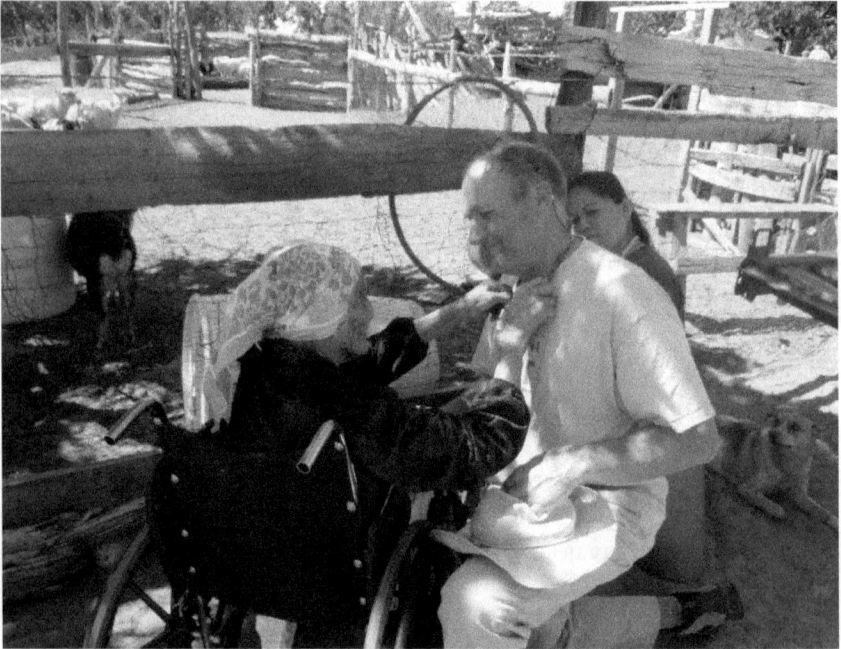

Berna Little gifting her personal necklace.

2008

The mission shuttle served people and animals mostly sheep, goats, cattle, horses, dogs and cats in five areas around the Navajo Nation. We worked in the New Mexico, Arizona, and Utah portions of the reservation. But, our favorite area was Navajo Mountain. In time we earned the friendship of **Hank and Francis Stevens**. Hank worked for the largest employer on the reservation, Peabody Coal, and Francis worked at the school for the second largest employer, the United States government.

Hank and Francis raised their family on Navajo Mountain but like most other Navajo families their children had to leave the reservation for higher education and better job opportunities. When Hank retired and the children moved away they sort of adopted us, and hosted us at their compound below Navajo Mountain on Piute Canyon road. The women on the mission would sleep indoors with running water and bath rooms, but the men on mission would sleep in a hogan outdoors. What an incredible experience to awake each morning viewing sunrise in the cool high desert air.

Hank loved to share his humble Navajo upbringing with the teams. He would walk us out to a small cedar tree near his house that used to be his home when he was young. He was raised on a blanket under this tree. When he got a little older his mother gave him away to another family off the reservation so that he could get a proper education. Many Navajo children never return after they leave the reservation, but after his education Hank returned to Navajo Mountain to care for his family. Hank and Francis are still caring for the elder Navajo. They are big workers at and supporters of Pioneer Day, they install water and waste systems for elderly homes, they provide leadership in the community, and they encourage and support the annual return of the "Christian Veterinarians."

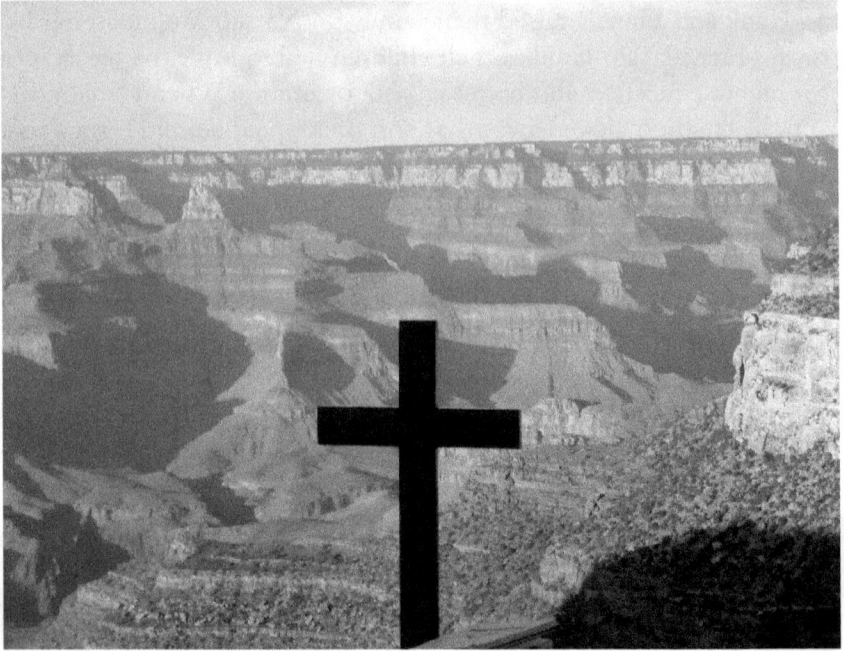

Each Year

On Sunday each year we visited the Grand Canyon which borders the Navajo Nation on the western side. Sunset over the canyon is a peaceful, awe-inspiring manifestation of God's great creative power. Most years we visited Monument Valley and Canyon De Chelly also. When at Navajo Mountain we would rush to the Piute Canyon "Rim" each evening to view the sunset. I don't want to make it sound like we just drove out, visited the scenery, and listened to stories. We were very intentional about meeting the stated goals of the mission listed at the beginning of this discourse. We set up clinics in numerous areas of the reservation. We enjoyed great relationships with amazing people in all of these locations. There are too many special people to mention in a book of this scope. While on mission, we visited shut-ins, led worship services, mentored young people, had twice-daily open devotionals, and, of course, provided care for thousands of various animals. In some years, we "vetted" over 3,000 animals, but we weren't dwelling on the animal count. It was the relationships that counted!

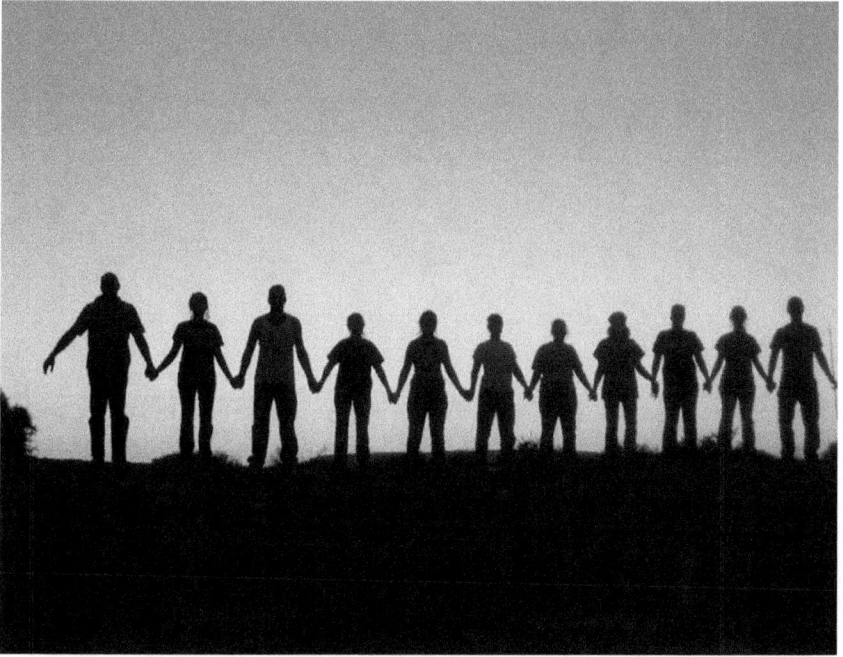

On the Piute Canyon Rim

CHAPTER 43
Cancer Therapy with a Cow Connection

In 2011 I agreed to re-enter the dairy business with a partner who was a longtime friend and client. David was a successful businessman, a visionary, and an honest man. I held immense respect for him and learned much through our association. He convinced me to join him in the dairy venture by allowing me to set the enterprise up any way I wanted. Together we built a business that we named Agri-Science Opportunities.

We were guided by a verse from the Old Testament book of Proverbs, which stated, "Where there is no vision, the people perish." Our vision for the enterprise was to have five different operating centers. One center was the "Production Center" where we managed the milking cows. A second center was the "Value Added Center" where we made great cheeses. A third center was the "Genetic Center" where we performed advanced reproductive techniques to multiply our best genetics. A fourth center was the "Education Center" where we partnered with veterinary schools, high schools, and grade schools to educate them about advanced reproductive techniques, modern agriculture, and where our food comes from. The final center was the "Innovation Center" where we performed research on animal and human maladies.

It was in the 'Innovation Center" that we happened upon a unique chemical with a cow connection that effectively killed cancer cells. Let me provide some background information about this unique chemical. My dairy business partner, David, had just lost a significant other to lung cancer, and after going through the grieving process, he returned to work intent on finding a cure for lung cancer. When he approached me with this new goal, I cautioned him not to make this his life's purpose.

Although he was quite a visionary, he was 75 years old, and his background was in real estate. I told him that there were hundreds of researchers with numerous degrees behind their names working on cancer cures every day who hadn't yet found the cure for lung cancer. He agreed, but nonetheless, he was going to try to find a cure himself, regardless of the circumstances.

He set out scouring the internet for lung cancer information every night. He would print out and bring to the farm many articles over the next weeks, asking my opinion on them. Nothing noteworthy really jumped out at me until the day he brought in an article that described an 80% decrease in lung cancer risk in dairymen (1).

When he asked my opinion on this article, I said it must be an aberrant occurrence, but I would investigate the findings. In my exploration, I found that identical results had been demonstrated in three different countries by different researchers. With this in mind, we initiated our own informal survey of various "long-timers" in the dairy industry and concluded for ourselves that dairymen could indeed have 80% or less risk of lung cancer compared to the general population. Our little survey did not identify any dairymen who had died of lung cancer.

We looked deeper into published research and found that dairymen with more cows showed lower risk than smaller herd owners, and that there was not even increased risk for dairymen who smoked. Another notable finding was that the reduced cancer risk did not extend to other livestock producers such as poultry, beef, or pork producers. We theorized that the reason only dairymen benefitted from reduced cancer risk was that dairymen were the only livestock producers who were intimate (touched them all) with all their animals every day, at least two times per day all year around. This meant that dairymen were constantly in the cow's space; able to inhale whatever the cow was putting into the atmosphere. By the way, the only cancer that has a reduced risk in dairymen is lung cancer which led us to believe the beneficial chemical was inhaled.

While I was investigating the original article showing the reduced lung cancer rate in dairymen; my partner continued to search the internet for other cancer related topics pertaining to cows. He came to me puzzled because there were almost no references to cancer in cattle. This was the first time that I really appreciated the fact that cows don't suffer from spontaneous cancers like other mammals. Cows really only suffer from squamous cell cancer in the eye and bovine lymphosarcoma in the hemic-lymphatic system. These cancers are not cancers resulting from spontaneous mutations of cells as in other animals. They are caused by external forces.

Cancer eye is caused by excessive solar radiation in cows with unpigmented eye tissues and it can be prevented by solar protection or genetically breeding cattle with pigmented skin around their eyes (Black Angus). Bovine lymphosarcoma is caused by a virus and can be controlled by testing and removal of affected carriers. Also of note is the fact that several other species appear to have no spontaneous cancers such as sheep, goats, deer, and antelopes. These animals are all of the ruminant classification, and this is noteworthy because I have a degree (MS) in ruminant nutrition.

How ruminants are able to resist spontaneous cancers and how they are able to transfer this resistance to dairymen grew to be the most important questions. For those not familiar, the outstanding characteristic of ruminants is their fermentative digestive system. Ruminants, in contrast to simple stomach animals (monogastrics), have a multi-compartment stomach that ferments feeds, and as a result, the bugs (bacteria and protozoa) in the rumen compartment produce many complex molecules. For example, cows do not have a requirement for 20 amino acids, or, three essential fatty acids, or multiple B vitamins in their diet like us monogastrics (simple stomach animals).

In the ruminants, these complex molecules are all made by "bugs" in the rumen. Our theory was that in the process of making these essential dietary components, the "bugs" also were making molecules that were heretofore not known. The heretofore unknown substance had the ability to kill cancer cells before the cells could grow into tumors. The substance could perhaps be eructated (burped) into the atmosphere where dairymen would inhale it, and receive protection in their lungs. In the ruminant, the unknown substance could also be absorbed into the bloodstream and protect the host animal from spontaneous cancers; killing cancer cells before they could become dangerous tumors.

Owing to our knowledge of ruminant physiology we postulated that the cancer-killing substance was an analogue of a B vitamin. We searched the internet and scientific literature, and in time, identified a molecule that we desired to pursue. It was actually being researched by an individual at a company in Ohio. The compound was called nitrosyl-cobalamine (NoCBL) which is a nitrous oxide (NO) carrying analog of vitamin B-12. Over the ensuing three years, we collaborated with the company and helped to obtain a pre-IND (Investigational New Drug) meeting with the Food and Drug Administration (FDA). We also manufactured the compound commercially in a North Carolina pharmaceutical lab, meeting all FDA guidelines.

At this point I will summarize some of our findings, but I have included citations of scientific references at the end of this book for those wishing for more details. Several studies demonstrated that NoCBL had amazing abilities against cancer (2, 3). It killed many types of cancer in nude mice test subjects. It also blocked the cancer cell survival mechanism in many cancer types making them susceptible to commonly used chemotherapies specific for those cancer types (4).

The cancer-killing properties of NoCBL were found to be modulated through its "Trojan Horse" nature. The body's cellular membrane receptors cannot distinguish NoCBL from normal B-vitamin, so it allows the compound inside the cell. Once inside, the nitrosyl (NO) moiety separates from the Cobalamin, and as a free radical causes damage to cell processes killing the cancer. It is true that all cells have free radical scavenging systems, but cancer cells have hundreds of times more B-12 receptors than normal cells. The normal cells take up very little NoCBL so, their scavenging systems handle the free radicals. However the cancer cells take up so much more NoCBL that it becomes a lethal dose (5).

Duke University Cancer Institute heard about our work and contacted us wanting to research this novel new therapy, because of its unique mode of action. However, before we could make all of the arrangements to test the novel product on Duke's cancer xenographs David passed away, and Agri-Science Opportunities had to be closed to satisfy his heirs. The result was that all work on NoCBL stopped.

My hope is that the work on this potentially life-changing product can be resurrected. I would like to see more product made and tested on Duke's xenographs. I would like to see if we can find NoCBL in the bloodstream or cells of a ruminant to confirm its role in spontaneous cancer prevention in ruminants. An amazing point is this: if this novel compound acts in humans like it appears to act in ruminants, it will not only be a cancer treatment, but it will be the first cancer prevention on the market. Eight billion people would potentially benefit.

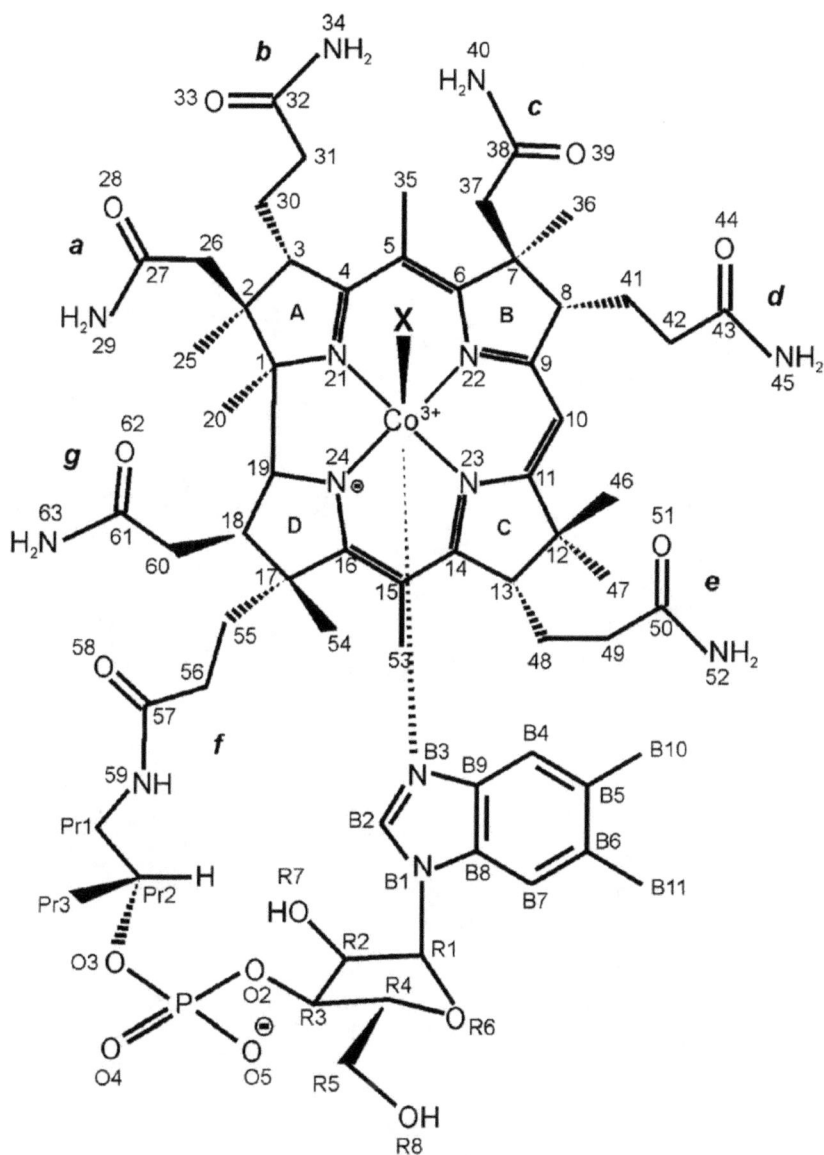

Labeling scheme for cobalamins. X = Me, Ado, H 2 O, CN, NO, NH 3 , NO 2 , SO 3 etc. NMR spectroscopy and molecular modelling studies of nitrosylcobalamin: Further evidence that the deprotonated, base-off form is important for nitrosylcobalamin in solution - Scientific Figure on ResearchGate. Available from: https://www.researchgate.net/figure/Labeling-scheme-for-cobalamins-X-Me-Ado-H-2-O-CN-NO-NH-3-NO-2-SO-3-etc_fig1_23720577 [accessed 25 Jan, 2024]

CHAPTER 44
Old-timer's (Alzheimer's) Research

The "Innovation Center" at Agri-Science Opportunities was also involved with a drug being developed for human Alzheimer's disease. In the process of working with the potential cancer treatment, Nitrosylcobalamin, and performing due diligence on our processes; we hired an outside consultant named Dr. John. He gave us a very thorough evaluation and a constructive critique. Two years later Dr. John returned to the Agri-Science farm offices with an urgent request. He knew we fiddled with drug development, and he needed help funding a new Alzheimer's disease treatment candidate.

I looked at the science behind the drug and decided to invest a few of my own funds to get this product under our control. Additionally, I convinced my partner David and his friends to invest. With our help Dr. John licensed this drug from another pharmaceutical company which had abandoned it. He then established a company to be responsible for the drug and incorporated it as T3D Pharmaceuticals in the year 2013. The drug is identified as T3D-959 and is aimed at improving glucose metabolism in the brain. T3D's scientists believe that aberrant glucose metabolism is responsible for the brain changes which ultimately lead to memory loss in Alzheimer's disease. They refer to this as "type 3 diabetes" and named the company T3D to symbolize their "type 3 diabetes" focus.

Over a period of 10-plus years T3D has continued to work toward FDA (Food and Drug Administration) approval of the drug for use in treating Alzheimer's disease. The process began with animal studies that verified the drug was able to cross through the blood-brain barrier, the body's neurological system protection mechanism. The safety of the drug was also established during the animal tests. We additionally observed some efficacy against animal Alzheimer's disease in the test animals.

In June 2015, T3D received its IND (investigational new drug) status from the FDA. This is the pivotal step in proving a new treatment! This status is required to test pharmaceuticals in human patients. At last, we were permitted to use the drug on people in Phase 2 trials. In these trials we established the drug's safety in people, established an effective dosage, and, as an incidental observation, noted some astounding efficacy in patients. There were numerous testimonials written to the T3D Company by patient caregivers and loved ones, which really encouraged us during these early trials. These were hand-written letters with heartfelt comments, and one is attached below. I hope you take the time and effort to read this note. There is a typed iteration that follows.

(Typed iteration)
Noted changes: by wife after two weeks in trial.
1. Much more alert and aware of surroundings
2. Much more engaged in conversation at home and in public

3. Critical of my driving. Aware of every changing light and tried to direct me how to go, when to stop and go. Critical of other drivers... commented on other drivers' traffic violations, etc.

4. Without prompting, went outside to repair Polaris (pool cleaner) that had disconnected from pool wall. Got the necessary tools without asking where they were located.

5. Started dispensing vitamins at breakfast. He did this on a daily basis for a number of years but quit 6-8 months ago. Now routine has resumed.

6. At my daughter's house in Charlotte, he asked if anyone would like a glass of wine. He got the wine he had chilled earlier, got the wine opener, and opened the wine. He then served it. For the last year or more, he has not remembered where he chilled the wine nor where the wine opener was kept. He also has not remembered how to operate my daughter's wine opener for the last year or more. He asked for <u>no</u> assistance when using it after the trial.

7. He has been choosing his clothes to wear without asking for advice.

8. He packed his suitcase (twice) without assistance. He has needed assistance with this task for at least one and a half to two years.

Getting drug approval has been a slow, laborious process slowed further by two years of Covid 19 delays because we were working with very high Covid risk patients. In mid-2022, we were allowed by the FDA to restart the phase two trials. Phase two trials were completed in early 2023 and the data is now analyzed. The T3D Company has shared preliminary Phase 2 conclusions with shareholders and the data looks very good.

T3D was selected to present its Phase 2 Topline Research Results at the 2023 (16th) Clinical Trials on Alzheimer's Disease Conference (CTAD). The presentation generated tremendous industry interest. We are now awaiting the FDA's end of Phase 2 meeting for a roadmap of requirements for the Phase 3 trial. The hope is that a large pharmaceutical company will review our data and the Phase 3 requirements, and purchase T3D so they can run the Phase 3 trials and market the product. T3D is too small to take the product all the way to market at this time. It has no distribution channels and it will probably require $200 million more for the completion of all aspects of market approval and distribution. More information can be obtained at the T3D website: http://www.t3dtherapeutics.com

Working with this potential Alzheimer's treatment has been an exhilarating roller-coaster ride. Several times during the 10-plus years of drug testing, we were delayed in progress or were out of funds. Miraculously we were able to overcome the obstacles and secure additional funds when they were needed. Why does all this matter? Alzheimer's disease is the sixth largest killer of adults over 65 years of age, and as people live longer these days, the cost of care for future Alzheimer's patients is predicted to be the number one drain on the United States healthcare system.

Today the healthcare industry is solving disease problems holistically with a "One Medicine" approach. "One Medicine" refers to the united efforts of all healthcare professionals, not just physicians. The above examples show that anyone with medical training should not sell short their potential. One may be able to help improve the quality of life for millions.

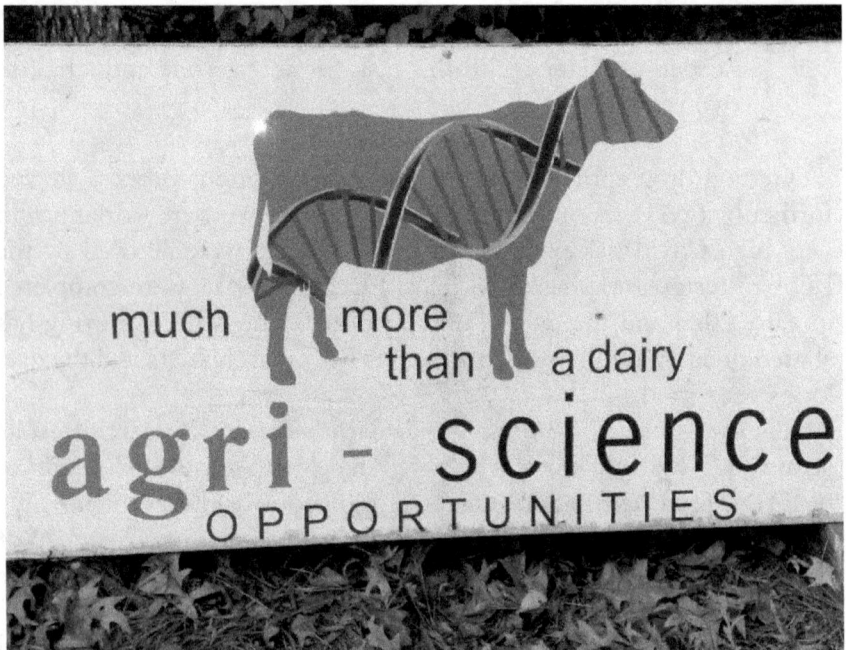

much more than a dairy
agri - science
OPPORTUNITIES

REFERENCES

Mastrangelo G, Grange JM, Fadda E, Fedeli U, Buja A, Lange JH.; Lung cancer risk: effect of dairy farming and the consequence of removing that occupational exposure. Am J Epidemiol. 2005 Jun 1;161(11):1037-46.

Bauer JA, Frye G, Bahr A, Gieg J, Brofman P.; Anti-tumor effects of nitrosylcobalamin against spontaneous tumors in dogs. Invest New Drugs. 2010;28:694–702.

Bauer JA, Morrison BH, Grane RW, et al.; Effects of interferon beta on transcobalamin II-receptor expression and antitumor activity of Nitrosylcobalamin. J Natl Cancer Inst. 2002;94:1010–1019.

Bauer JA, Lupica JA, Schmidt H, et al.; Nitrosylcobalamin potentiates the anti-neoplastic effects of chemotherapeutic agents via suppression of survival signaling. PLoS ONE. 2007;2:e1313.

Dunphy, Michael; Sysel, Annette; Lupica, Joseph; Griffith, Kristie; Sherrod, Taylor; ... [+]A Stability-Indicating HPLC Method for the Determination of Nitrosylcobalamin (NO-Cbl), a Novel Vitamin B12 Analog. Chromatographia, Volume 77 (8) – Mar 14, 2014.

ABOUT THE AUTHOR

Dr. Sam Galphin grew up in a rural community in South Carolina, cultivated by a farmer and mixed animal veterinarian father and nurtured by a loving schoolteacher mother. He developed deep fondness for agriculture, where less than one percent of the population is active in food production. He believes that agriculture is key to the sustainability of humanity.

Dr. Galphin's college years at Clemson University (BS) and the University of Georgia (DVM) reinforced a growing passion for feeding people when studies of food insecurity and simultaneous explosive population growth seemed to threaten humanity's future. He chose a veterinary career to elevate his opportunities for increasing food availability. It was not the usual veterinary career that most Americans see, but the distinctly different field of food supply veterinarian medicine. Except for a stint in the United States Air Force, his entire adult employment has involved agriculture and food production.

Dr. Galphin had no real career template to follow in his food supply veterinary calling, so he made his own way. After analyzing the food animal industries, he formulated the philosophy, "If I can make an economically significant change in a food animal facility, I can increase food production through profits." He devised a training program to prepare him for his chosen career and create a demand for his skills. He specialized in reproduction, emphasized the epidemiology of diseases, and enrolled in a nutrition degree program while teaching veterinary medicine at Mississippi State University (MS). As a type of post-graduate education, he later operated several dairies of his own.

Much of this book reports the daily adventures and challenges of food supply veterinary medicine delivery in numerous southeastern states and many foreign countries as demand for Dr. Galphin's services escalated. Then, in mid-career, came another calling, this one from the

Creator. He gained the opportunity to mentor and be mentored by hundreds of faithful young people as they accompanied him into the mission field for almost thirty years. The veterinary mission shuttles allowed him to take his unique approach to food production to the world's poorer communities and help build a heart for service in these young aspiring professionals. The missions assisted with both physical and spiritual needs and introduced him to many special people around the globe.

Along the way, Dr. Galphin delved into finding solutions for animal and human diseases. The culmination of these efforts will be the soon anticipated marketing of a treatment for Alzheimer's disease and perhaps the development of a cancer treatment with a cow connection!